Osteoporosis

A Guide to
Prevention & Treatment

John F. Aloia, MD
Winthrop-University Hospital

Leisure Press
Champaign, Illinois

Developmental Editor: Lisa Busjahn
Managing Editor: Holly Gilly
Copyeditor: Bruce Owens
Proofreader: Steve Otto
Production Director: Ernie Noa
Typesetter: Cindy Pritchard
Text Design: Keith Blomberg
Text Layout: Tara Welsch
Cover Design: Jack Davis
Illustrations By: Ranee Rogers
Printed By: Versa Press

ISBN: 0-88011-354-5

Library of Congress Cataloging-in-Publication Data

Aloia, John F.
  Osteoporosis : a guide to prevention and treatment.

  Bibliography: p.
  Includes index.
  1. Osteoporosis--Prevention. 2. Osteoporosis--
Treatment. I. Title.
RC931.073A43 1989   616.7'16   88-13819
ISBN 0-88011-354-5

Printed in the United States of America

10 9 8 7 6 5 4 3 2

Leisure Press
A Division of Human Kinetics
  Publishers, Inc.
Box 5076, Champaign, IL
  61825-5076
1-800-747-4457

UK Office:
Human Kinetics Publishers (UK)
  Ltd.
P.O. Box 18
Rawdon, Leeds LS19 6TG
England
(0532) 504211

Contents

Preface   ix

Acknowledgments   xi

CHAPTER 1: OSTEOPOROSIS AND CALCIUM   **1**
  Who Develops Osteoporosis   1
  What is Calcium Homeostasis?   2
  Calcium Homeostasis and Body Systems   2
  Calcium Homeostasis and the Endocrine System   4
  Measuring Calcium Balance   7
  Summary   7

CHAPTER 2: THE HEALTHY SKELETAL SYSTEM AND
OSTEOPOROSIS   **9**
  Skeletal Tissue   10
  Bone Cells and Remodeling   12
  Bones as Organs   14
  Bone Gain and Bone Loss   19
  Osteoporosis Classification   23
  Summary   25

CHAPTER 3: OSTEOPOROSIS RISK FACTORS   **27**
  Modifiable and Nonmodifiable Risk Factors   27
  The Influence of Heredity on Peak Bone Mass   28
  The Effects of Inactivity and Activity on Bone Mass   29
  The Effects of Nutrition on Bone Mass   30
  Estrogen's Effect on Bone Mass   31
  Other Hormones' Effects on Bone Mass   33
  Cigarette Smoking's Effects on Bone Mass   34
  The Effects of Drugs and Illnesses on Bone Mass   34
  An Osteoporosis Risk Quiz and Prevention Commandments 35
  Factors Influencing Bone Strength   37
  Reduced Bone Strength   37
  Summary   38

CHAPTER 4: AVOIDING OSTEOPOROTIC INJURIES   **41**
Risks for Tripping and Falling in the Elderly   43
How to Avoid Tripping and Falling   46
How to Avoid Injury to the Spine   48
A Lifelong Strategy for Preventing Osteoporotic Fractures   51
Summary   51

CHAPTER 5: OSTEOPOROSIS AND THE CALCIUM CRAZE   **53**
What Is the Calcium Craze?   54
The Evidence for Increasing Dietary Intake of Calcium   55
What About Calcium Supplements?   57
Which Calcium Supplement Is Best?   58
What is Elemental Calcium?   64
Calcium Supplements and Bioavailability   65
Should Calcium Supplements Contain Other Minerals and
    Vitamins?   66
When Should Calcium Supplements Be Taken?   67
Can Calcium Supplementation Be Harmful?   67
Summary   69

**CHAPTER 6: PREVENTING OSTEOPOROSIS THROUGH
PROPER NUTRITION**   **71**
New American Dietary Goals   71
Dietary Guidelines   72
Estimating Calcium Intake   80
How to Increase Calcium Intake   86
The U.S. RDA and Nutrition Labeling   95
Achieving an Adequate Calcium Intake   97
Other Dietary Factors and Osteoporosis   100
Vegetarian and Weight-Loss Diets   105
Summary   107
Appendix: Daily Menus for 1,200-, 1,500-,
    1,800-Calorie/1,500-Milligram Calcium Diets   109

CHAPTER 7: THE ESTROGEN CONTROVERSY   **115**
What Is the Estrogen Controversy?   115
The Benefits of Estrogen Treatment   116
The Potential Risks of Estrogen Treatment   118
Medications Used in Estrogen-Replacement Therapy   121
The Role of Progestins in Estrogen-Replacement Therapy   123
Aggressive Versus Conservative Menopause Management   125
Suggestions for Recommending Treatment Options   128
Summary   129

CHAPTER 8: EXERCISING FOR SKELETAL HEALTH   **131**
Aerobic and Strengthening Exercises   132
Four Components of an Effective Exercise Program   134
Exercise Recommendations for Skeletal Health   134
A Home Gym Preventive Exercise Program   137
Physical Training for the Elderly   146
Exercise Recommendations for Osteoporotic Women   147
A Home Osteoporosis Exercise Program   147
Summary   155

CHAPTER 9: DIAGNOSTIC TESTING   **157**
Bone Mass Measurement   157
Radiographic Morphometry   158
Total Body Neutron Activation Analysis and Whole-Body
    Counting   158
Single-Photon Absorptiometry   159
Dual-Photon Absorptiometry   159
Computed Tomography   162
Answers to Questions About Densitometry   162
Other Tests Used in Evaluating and Treating Osteoporosis   168
Summary   173

CHAPTER 10: REHABILITATIVE TREATMENT STRATEGIES   **175**
Rehabilitation Goals for Osteoporosis   175
Treatment Immediately Following Vertebral Fracture   176
Rehabilitative Treatment of Vertebral Fractures   177
Avoiding Future Vertebral Fractures   180
Psychological Adjustments to Osteoporosis and Fractures   180
Summary   183

CHAPTER 11: TREATMENT OF PAIN FROM OSTEOPOROSIS   **185**
The Causes of Chronic Pain   185
A Multiple-Front Approach to Treating Chronic Pain   186
Uses of Drugs in Pain Treatment   187
Uses of Other Modalities for Pain Treatment   189
Treatment of Pain Due to Muscle Spasms   190
Who Should Attend a Pain Clinic?   190
Summary   191

CHAPTER 12: DRUG THERAPY FOR OSTEOPOROSIS   **193**
Characteristics of Ideal Drug Therapy   194
Classification of New Drug Treatments   195
Drugs That Reduce Bone Resorption   196

Drugs That Increase Bone Formation 199
Combination Drug Therapy 200
Sequential Drug Therapy 200
Drugs that Increase Calcium Absorption 201
Who Should Undergo Drug Therapy? 201
Summary 202
Appendix: Instructions for the Injection of Calcitonin 203

CHAPTER 13: HOPE FOR THE FUTURE **211**
Current Research in Osteoporosis 212
Future Research—What Does the Next Decade Hold? 215

Glossary 217

References 227

Index 231

About the Author 236

Preface

As many as 20 million Americans suffer from osteoporosis, a disease that decreases the mass of bones and increases their fragility. Annual costs for medical treatment range between 7 and 10 billion dollars. For Americans over the age of 44, osteoporosis is a contributing cause in 1.3 million fractures a year. Because the effects of aging weaken the skeleton, especially in postmenopausal women, the risk for fractures increases with age.

The U.S. Bureau of the Census has estimated that by the year 2050, 21.7% of the American population will be older than 65, a figure nearly double that of 11.4% in 1981. The economic impact of potentially twice as many hip fractures in 2050 as in 1981 is hard to imagine. Yet the true toll of osteoporosis is perhaps most meaningfully measured in personal terms. Though osteoporosis is not a killer—most women who have the disease die from other causes—it is often debilitating. Six months after a hip fracture only 25% of patients are fully recovered, 50% are in need of assistance with activities of daily living, and 25% require nursing home care. Osteoporosis often leads to pain, disability, and depression. Governmental and private health agencies, researchers, clinicians, and the general public must work together to develop strategies to prevent and treat osteoporosis.

Recognizing these challenges led me to join the osteoporosis research team headed by Stanton H. Cohn, PhD, at Brookhaven National Laboratory in Upton, New York. My research, conducted over two decades, has been based on the belief that understanding the causes of low bone mass would eventually lead to osteoporosis prevention. In the last decade, I established the Osteoporosis Diagnosis and Treatment Center at Winthrop University Hospital in Mineola, New York. Developments on the cutting edge of osteoporosis research at Brookhaven and Winthrop have been made available to hundreds of women in the region. Research advances have also occurred at a phenomenal rate elsewhere in the U.S. and abroad.

In 1984, the National Institutes of Health held a consensus conference on osteoporosis. Consensus meetings bring experts together to provide the best advice for public health policy from the available information on a topic. After the conference, the consensus findings were disseminated to the public. Less than 3 years later (February 1987), the National Institutes of Health cosponsored a meeting with the National Osteoporosis Foundation called "Research Directions in Osteoporosis." Scientists were brought together from the United States and Europe to present recent findings relevant to osteoporosis. Important information had been gathered since the 1984 consensus conference.

The information confirmed that osteoporosis is a preventable disorder and affects many women. Yet, until the last few years, when we told a woman that she suffered a fracture of the spine as a result of osteoporosis, frequently neither she nor her daughter was familiar with the term. This situation has improved greatly as a result of recent media attention. The first voluntary organization devoted to reducing the impact of osteoporosis, the National Osteoporosis Foundation, was founded in 1985.

An informational public survey was carried out in 1982 and again in 1984 by the founding members of the National Osteoporosis Foundation. It showed that public awareness of osteoporosis had grown as a result of media attention. However, 40% of women were still unaware of the disease, most women had not acted on the basis of their recently acquired knowledge, and only 38% were aware of the role of calcium in helping to prevent osteoporosis. Only 10% of women had learned about osteoporosis from their physicians, and only 4% had asked their physicians about osteoporosis. Thus, despite scientific advances, public education concerning osteoporosis requires more effort.

A major purpose of *Osteoporosis: A Guide to Prevention and Treatment* is to provide women with current information that shows osteoporosis to be both preventable and treatable. In addition, current information about osteoporosis is important for a broad range of health professionals, including dietitians, nurses, physical therapists, physicians, pharmacists, and social workers. It is my hope that each of these practitioners benefits by learning about osteoporosis and that a team effort can be mounted to combat it.

Acknowledgments

The author would like to acknowledge the specific contributions of the following: my wife Vera for her patience; Mary Greaney for secretarial support; Lynn Chimon, M.S., R.D., for contributions on nutrition; Virginia Dittko, R.N., M.A., for contributions on Calcitonin injections; and David Faegenberg, M.D., for providing X-ray material.

1 CHAPTER

Osteoporosis and Calcium

Osteoporosis has recently become almost a household word. Even if you don't have osteoporosis, you probably have an older relative who has broken a bone following a fall, and all of us are familiar with the sight of an older woman who is bent over as a result of osteoporosis. Still, most people can't define osteoporosis. What is this disabling disease that is so common in older women?

Osteoporosis is a condition in which the amount of bone tissue is so low that the bones easily fracture in response to minimal force. A person with osteoporosis can fracture a wrist or hip from a fall on the ice or receive a broken rib from an affectionate hug. Bending at the waist to pick up a grandchild may be accompanied by excruciating back pain as a result of a spinal fracture. In fact, the amount of bone tissue may be so low that a person fractures the spine simply by carrying the weight of the body.

WHO DEVELOPS OSTEOPOROSIS?

Women are the most likely to suffer osteoporotic fractures. Approximately 20% of women develop spinal fractures, and fractures of the *humerus*,* ribs, and pelvis are also common in women. A study of fractures at the Mayo Clinic in Rochester, Minnesota (Melton & Riggs, 1983), revealed that 33% of women and 17% of men who live to be 90 suffer a hip fracture and 24% of women and 5% of men break their wrist (Colles' fracture). Children are also subject to wrist fractures, which occur more frequently at a younger age than other types of osteoporotic fractures, reaching a plateau at around age 60 in women.

Most other fractures continue to increase in incidence (the number of new fractures per year) through old age. Women in their 60s

---

*Italicized words appear in the glossary at the end of the book.

are most prone to spinal fractures, whereas those in their 70s and 80s are more likely to fracture the *femur*.

Osteoporosis is a major health threat to the elderly. Fortunately, it is both preventable and treatable. This chapter and the next outline some basic biological facts you need to grasp in understanding how osteoporosis can be successfully prevented and treated.

WHAT IS CALCIUM HOMEOSTASIS?

The body must be able to react to changes in the external environment while keeping its own internal environment intact. The internal environment must remain relatively unchanged to maintain an optimal environment for the function of cells. The checks and balances that constantly act to maintain the optimal internal environment are referred to as *homeostasis*, which means "keeping things the same." Calcium homeostasis involves the numerous influences that maintain the blood calcium level in an optimal range for cellular function. When the internal environment is in an optimal state, one is healthy. But if homeostasis is disrupted, a disease is said to be present. Osteoporosis results from changes in calcium homeostasis and is categorized as a disorder of bone metabolism.

Living things are organized as cells, tissues, organs, and systems. Cells are the smallest units of living matter. Tissues consist of the same type of cells. Organs have specific functions and their own nerve and blood supplies. A system is a group of organs that perform similar functions or that work together to perform one complex function. The systems of the body work together so that the entire body functions harmoniously.

CALCIUM HOMEOSTASIS AND BODY SYSTEMS

Four systems are of particular importance in calcium homeostasis: gastrointestinal, urinary, skeletal, and endocrine. The skeletal system is frequently considered together with the muscles attached to it and is referred to as the musculoskeletal system.

The Gastrointestinal System

The digestive system processes food into a form that can enter the circulation. Stomach juices liquify food so it may easily pass into the small intestine. Absorption is the process whereby digested food first enters the cells in the lining of the small intestine and then enters the bloodstream to be transported throughout the body. The remaining waste products proceed to the large intestine and are emptied into the external environment through the stool.

Calcium enters the body through the diet and is absorbed into the circulation from the small intestine. The movement of a substance into or out of cells is referred to as *transport*. Calcium absorption occurs by two processes, active transport and passive transport. Active transport of calcium is a controlled (active) process that depends on the body's need for calcium. Calcium homeostasis is maintained by influencing the active transport of calcium. Passive transport, however, depends on the amount of calcium present in the diet. As more calcium is ingested, more will be absorbed through passive transport. Ordinarily, an adult woman absorbs only about one third of the calcium she eats.

The Urinary System

The urinary system filters blood and eliminates waste products. It also conserves water, sodium, calcium, potassium, phosphorus, protein, and glucose. Impurities are filtered out by the kidneys, and the substances that are useful to the body are reabsorbed from the urine into the bloodstream.

The kidneys filter the calcium in the blood and allow some calcium to be lost in the urine. Ordinarily, on an average calcium intake, less than 150 milligrams of calcium per day is found in the urine. An excess of calcium in the urine is called *hypercalciuria*. The kidneys act as an escape route for excess calcium. If too much calcium is absorbed from the diet, it can be removed from the circulation by the kidneys and passed out of the body through the urine.

The Skeletal System

Almost all the calcium (99%) in the body is stored in bone. One usually thinks of bone as static, but it is an active tissue that is continually changing, or *remodeling*. Bone is continuously broken down (*resorption*) and reformed (formation), even in old age. If an inadequate amount of calcium is entering the circulation from the intestine or if an excess of calcium is lost through the urine, bone will be resorbed to maintain the level of calcium in the blood.

The movement of calcium may be influenced in each of three target organs (intestines, kidney, and bone) independently of the others. For example, intestinal surgery may result in lowered calcium absorption, *thiazide* diuretics ("water pills") may decrease calcium loss in the urine, and exercise may increase bone formation. The kidney is limited in the amount of calcium it can conserve and the intestine in the amount of dietary calcium it can absorb, but bone has a seemingly endless reservoir of calcium. Bone is the skeletal "bank" from which calcium may be "withdrawn" for homeostasis if needed. The skeletal bank is always open—it is like a cash machine where you can withdraw or deposit money 24 hours a day. Unfortunately, if withdrawals keep exceeding deposits, the amount of calcium in the skeletal bank decreases, and the skeleton becomes susceptible to fracture.

CALCIUM HOMEOSTASIS AND THE ENDOCRINE SYSTEM

Endocrine glands produce, store, and secrete hormones into the circulation. The hormones are then carried to another part of the body to help control the rate of chemical reaction. The distant organ on which a hormone acts is its target organ.

The *endocrine system* consists of the hypothalamus, pituitary gland, thyroid, pancreas, parathyroid, thymus, adrenal glands, and gonads. Each of these organs is important in maintaining homeostasis. The three hormones that control calcium homeostasis are called the *calciotropic hormones*. Other hormones, such as growth hormone and *estrogen*, may have important effects on the skeleton, but their influence on calcium homeostasis is indirect.

The calciotropic hormones are *parathyroid hormone, calcitonin,* and *calcitriol* (the active form of vitamin D). These hormones help maintain blood calcium levels at an optimal level by influencing the transport of calcium between the circulation and the gastrointestinal tract, the kidney, and the skeleton.

Parathyroid Hormone

Parathyroid hormone is made by the four parathyroid glands, which are located in the neck on the thyroid gland. When the blood level of calcium decreases, secretion of parathyroid hormone increases, and when blood calcium is elevated, secretion of parathyroid hormone decreases.

If blood calcium levels become low, the parathyroid glands detect the change and secrete parathyroid hormone into the circulation. Parathyroid hormone increases bone resorption, resulting in an increase in blood calcium. The hormone increases the production of the active form of vitamin D, calcitriol, by the kidney, resulting in increased calcium absorption from the intestine into the circulation, and also acts on the kidneys so that less calcium is excreted into the urine. These effects on the three target organs result in blood calcium returning to normal.

Calcitonin

Calcitonin is a less potent hormone than is parathyroid hormone. It antagonizes, or counters, the effects of parathyroid hormone on bone. Calcitonin is manufactured in special cells of the thyroid gland. The major stimulus for the secretion of calcitonin into the bloodstream is a high blood calcium level, or *hypercalcemia*. Calcitonin decreases bone resorption and increases the urinary excretion of calcium.

Calcitriol

Vitamin D is not a hormone; it is, however, converted into an active form, calcitriol, that fits the definition of a hormone. Vitamin D is inactive by itself but enters the body in two ways: (a) by reaction of ultraviolet light with the skin and (b) through the food that is eaten. Vitamin D must be converted into its more active forms. This occurs first in the liver and then in the kidney. Calcitriol is secreted by the kidney into the circulation. It acts on the intestine to increase calcium absorption and on bone to increase bone resorption. The manufacture of calcitriol by the kidney is stimulated by several factors, including parathyroid hormone.

Gonadal Hormones

Although estrogen's primary function is not to maintain an optimal blood level of calcium, it profoundly affects the skeleton. Estrogen is manufactured in the ovaries, which produce an egg about once a month (in the middle of the menstrual cycle). The age at which the menstrual cycle begins is called *menarche* (usually between the ages of 10 and 14). *Progestins* (similar to *progesterone*) produced by the ovaries after ovulation stimulate a buildup of the lining of the uterus. If an egg is not fertilized, the levels of estrogens and progestins decline and the lining of the uterus is shed, resulting in *menstruation*. Change in the production of estrogens and progestins is controlled by two pituitary hormones called Follicle Stimulating Hormone (FSH) and Luteinizing Hormone (LH). In midlife (around age 50), the ovaries shrink in size, stop producing eggs, and produce progressively less hormonal products (estrogens and progestins). The cessation of menstruation is called *amenorrhea* (meaning "no menstruation"). When this occurs naturally in mid-life, it is referred to as *menopause*. The stage preceding menopause is sometimes referred to as *perimenopausal* and the years following the time menstruation has ceased for 1 year as postmenopausal.

Estrogens are responsible for the rapid growth of the skeleton in girls during puberty and for the eventual closure of the ends of long bones so that growth ceases. Estrogen deficiency during adolescence and early adulthood will result in the formation of a skeleton with less bone tissue.

In later life, estrogens antagonize the effect of parathyroid hormone on bone resorption. Estrogens do not have a direct effect on bone resorption but, rather, act indirectly by interfering with parathyroid hormone. Estrogens stimulate the formation of calcitriol by the kidney and may also stimulate calcitonin secretion. Thus, estrogens have multiple indirect effects that promote calcium retention in the body. Estrogen loss at menopause results in increased bone resorption and reduced calcium absorption.

In men, similar effects are observed with *testosterone*, a hormone produced in the testes. Testosterone stimulates growth, is responsible for the cessation of growth, and also decreases the adult's bone resorption.

Let us now look at how the calciotropic hormones act on their target organs to keep the blood calcium level in the normal, or optimal, range. Suppose that there is a very low intake of calcium in the diet, resulting in less calcium being absorbed and a slight decrease in blood levels of calcium. The parathyroid glands detect the lowering of blood calcium and secrete parathyroid hormone. The increase in parathyroid hormone secretion results in an increase in bone resorption that will not be counteracted by calcitonin because calcitonin secretion will decline. In addition, parathyroid hormone increases the synthesis of calcitriol. The higher levels of calcitriol increase absorption of calcium from the intestine. Parathyroid hormone also reduces the urinary excretion of calcium.

These processes will continue until the level of calcium in the blood returns to normal.

An important point is that this process occurs in total disregard of the effect on the target organs; that is, bone mass was sacrificed to maintain blood calcium levels in the optimal range. The loss of bone was an undesirable effect of a homeostatic mechanism. When excess calcium is lost to the environment or when sufficient calcium cannot be obtained from the environment, bone will be lost. If there is insufficient dietary calcium, a loss of calcium through the urine, or an inability to increase production of calcitriol so that calcium absorption cannot increase appropriately, parathyroid hormone will produce bone loss. This sequence of events occurs in old age because aged kidneys cannot generate sufficient calcitriol when the intake of dietary calcium is inadequate.

MEASURING CALCIUM BALANCE

Calcium homeostasis may be studied using the balance technique. This involves hospitalization in a special research unit, usually a clinical research center or a "metabolic ward." The amount of calcium in the diet, stool, and urine is carefully measured. The balance is the difference between the amount of calcium entering (through the diet) and the amount leaving the body (through the stool and urine). If the body retains calcium, the balance is said to be positive; if intake is equal to output, the balance is said to be zero; and if there is net loss of calcium from the body to the external environment, the balance is negative.

Because 99% of the body's calcium is in the skeleton, calcium balance actually reflects the gain and loss of bone. The difference between bone formation and bone resorption determines whether bone is lost or gained (or whether calcium balance is negative or positive). The gain and loss of bone in various stages of the life cycle will be discussed in chapter 2.

SUMMARY

Osteoporosis is a condition in which the amount of bone tissue is so low that the bones easily fracture in response to minimal force. Elderly women are most likely to suffer osteoporotic fractures of the wrist, femur, and spine. Recent research has indicated that osteoporosis is both preventable and treatable. To understand how this is so, you must first learn some rudimentary facts of biology.

Four systems work together to maintain an optimal level of blood calcium in the body: gastrointestinal, urinary, skeletal, and endocrine. The skeleton is being remodeled continuously, with bone being removed (resorption) and replaced (formation). Three calciotropic hormones promote calcium homeostasis: Parathyroid hormone increases bone resorption and the manufacture of calcitriol, calcitonin decreases bone resorption, and calcitriol increases calcium absorption. Estrogens are important in skeletal growth. During menopause, the loss of estrogens in the woman's body results in both increased sensitivity of bone to the effects of parathyroid hormone and accelerated bone loss.

The skeleton serves as a reservoir of calcium. If a person takes in an inadequate amount of calcium or if he or she loses an excessive amount to the environment, calcium is removed from bone to meet the body's needs. Calcium balance refers to the amounts of calcium entering and leaving the body. Equal amounts mean the balance is zero. Unfortunately, when calcium is continually withdrawn from the skeletal "bank" (negative balance), bone mass declines so much that the skeleton becomes at risk for osteoporotic fractures.

2 CHAPTER

The Healthy Skeletal System and Osteoporosis

Our bones are a marvelous feat of engineering. The skeleton allows us to move and protects our internal organs and bone marrow from injury. Bone must be both light and solid to allow movement and support our bodies. In addition, it has to be flexible so it can bend and change shape, rather than shatter, in response to strong forces. Certain diseases cause bone to soften (osteomalacia) or to harden and become brittle (osteosclerosis). Both of these diseases and osteoporosis increase the chance of fracture as we grow older.

In the adult, the structural function and shape of bone depends to a great extent on the stress placed on it. Bone adapts to the use we put it to—the more we mechanically load our bones, the more they will increase in volume or mass, and they do so specifically along the lines of mechanical loading. This adaptation is called *modeling.* In other words, the skeleton responds to stress by forming additional bone; when the load on the skeleton is reduced, bone mass decreases.

In chapter 1, I discussed bone's chemical function as a reservoir of calcium for the body's use. This function has a more ancient evolutionary origin than the purely mechanical function of locomotion and support. Animals required protection against accumulation of waste products and control of body minerals before the development of a hard skeleton. It is not surprising, then, that the chemical functions of bone have primacy over its structural functions. The body sacrifices a quantity of bone regardless of the mechanical stress placed on it if it needs the minerals in the bone for other purposes. This may explain why osteoporosis and osteoporotic fractures develop: Osteoporosis results when the body has not obtained an adequate amount of mineral from the environment and when the mechanical load is insufficient for development of new bone due to physical inactivity.

9

This chapter discusses bone at the three organizational levels of the skeletal system: tissue, cells, and organs.

SKELETAL TISSUE

The two types of skeletal tissue in bone are *cortical bone* and *trabecular bone* (see Figure 2.1). Cortical bone is densely packed, and comprises about 80% of all skeletal tissue. Cortical bone surrounds the trabecular bone, which is made up of intermeshing thin, bony plates that fill the bony cavities and are in contact with the bone marrow. Trabecular bone is influenced to a greater extent than is cortical bone by changes in skeletal metabolism. Different bones have different proportions of cortical and trabecular bone—for example, the long bones of the extremities are mainly cortical tissue, whereas the vertebral bodies have more trabecular mass. The relative proportion of trabecular bone increases, as does the incidence of fractures from osteoporosis, at the ends of the long bones.

Bone structure is a combination of matrix and mineral. The soft bone matrix consists primarily of *collagen* arranged in overlapping fibers that form spaces in the bone. These spaces are filled with crystals of calcium, phosphorus, and water. These crystals, or *hydroxyapatite*, give bone its strength, and the matrix allows it to bend

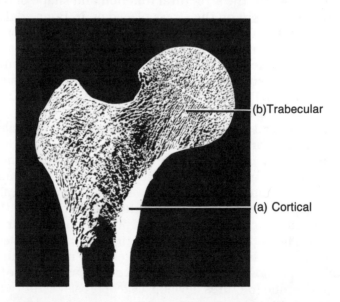

Figure 2.1 The two types of skeletal tissues are cortical (a) and trabecular (b). *Note.* From *A Colour Atlas of Bone Disease* (p. 35) by V. Parsons, 1980, London: Wolfe Medical. Adapted by permission.

rather than shatter under force. When new bone is formed, the soft matrix is deposited first, followed by the addition of bone mineral (hydroxyapatite). The process of depositing minerals in bone is referred to as *mineralization* or *calcification*.

Visualizing the bone matrix as a handkerchief may be helpful in understanding bone structure. A handkerchief can be stretched, folded, and pulled. Its flexibility allows it to sustain stress by changing shape, or bending. If the spaces between the threads of the handkerchief were filled with cement—just as the spaces in the matrix of a bone are filled with hydroxyapatite—the handkerchief would also have a strong, rigid structure.

In osteoporosis the composition of the bone matrix and hydroxyapatite is the same as that of normal, healthy bone, but there is less bone tissue (see Figure 2.2). Osteoporosis literally means "porous bone."

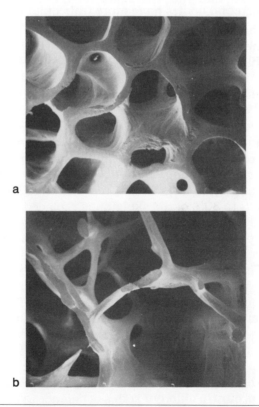

a

b

Figure 2.2   In osteoporosis the composition of bone matrix and hydroxyapatite is the same as that of normal, healthy bone (a), but there is less bone tissue (b). Micrographs courtesy of Dr. David Dempster with permission from the *Journal of Bone and Mineral Research*.

Diseases such as *osteomalacia*—which occurs when bone becomes softer as a result of an increased amount of unmineralized matrix—also result in an increased risk of fracture. In osteomalacia, however, the composition of the bone material changes. Osteoporosis and osteomalacia are *metabolic bone diseases*, which refers to generalized disease of the bone; that is, the entire skeleton is affected. In contrast, for example, a bone tumor affects only a localized part of the skeleton or a specific bone.

BONE CELLS AND REMODELING

The three types of bone cells are *osteoblasts*, *osteoclasts*, and *osteocytes*. Osteoblasts produce bone matrix, which, when mineral (primarily calcium and phosphate) is added, forms calcified bone. Osteoclasts break down calcified bone (resorption). Osteocytes are found within bone rather than on its surface and may begin the process of bone calcification.

In the last chapter, bone remodeling was discussed from the perspective of maintaining calcium homeostasis. Another purpose of bone remodeling is to replace older bone that has developed microscopic breaks, called microfractures, with new bone. Microfractures in bones are similar to the kinds of defects in the metal of airplane wings and bridge bolts that engineers are concerned with when those structures become old. Accumulation of microfractures can reduce the strength of bone.

The remodeling cycle lasts from 4 months to as long as 1 year. In an adult, 10% to 30% of the skeleton is replaced by remodeling each year. Remodeling occurs in the following way (see Figure 2.3). Osteoclasts appear and dissolve bone. The osteoclastic cells eventually die, leaving a hole in the bone. Osteocytes and osteoblasts then appear. The osteoblasts fill the hole with matrix, and the bone is mineralized. Unmineralized matrix is called osteoid. If the osteoblasts do not completely fill the hole, less bone is formed than is resorbed at that site. If the osteoblasts fill the hole with extra bone, then bone formation exceeds bone resorption. Remodeling balance is a term used to indicate whether extra bone was formed (positive balance) or less bone was formed (negative balance). At the end of this process, there is little cellular activity in the bone.

Remodeling occurs in different states of balance in different skeletal sites. Thus, in different parts of the skeleton, bone may be in the quiescent, the resorption, or the formation phases of this continuous cycle. Each site undergoing remodeling is referred to as a remodeling unit. There are over a million remodeling units in the

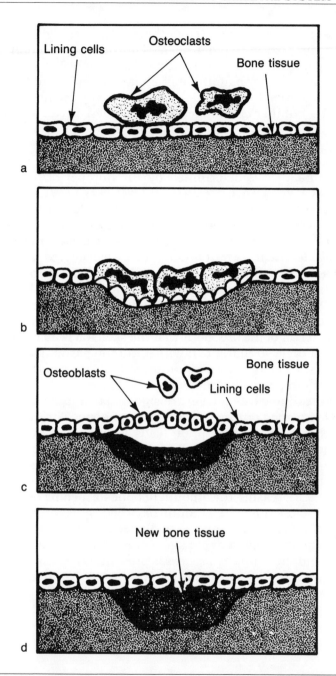

Figure 2.3 Bone remodeling cycle. Remodeling occurs when osteoclasts are activated (a) and dissolve bone (b). Osteoblasts later appear and fill the cavity with bone matrix which is then mineralized (c). The new bone is then in a quiescent phase (d).

skeleton at any given time—ten of these units together have only a volume the size of a pin's head. The process whereby bone remodeling begins is called activation. The number of remodeling units determines the magnitude of changes in skeletal (calcium) balance. In addition to mechanical stress, parathyroid hormone can increase the number of remodeling units whereas calcitonin may reduce the number. When overall calcium balance is measured, the sum of the balance of all the remodeling units determines whether calcium balance is positive or negative. The magnitude of change in calcium balance is determined by the number of remodeling units.

Many scientists believe that the local activation of remodeling units results from the generation of minute electrical currents at the sites of microfractures where bone is stressed by mechanical forces. The electrical current is detected by osteocytes which then transmit a signal to the cells lining the surface of bone. Osteoclasts then appear and begin to dissolve bone in the direction of the microfracture. Osteoblasts fill the hole with additional bone and there is then additional bone that can withstand increased mechanical forces. The result of the process is that the skeleton is able to change the shape of bone so that it can withstand the particular forces to which it is subjected. This adaptation of the shape of the bone to mechanical force is called modeling.

It is not clear how osteoblasts are signaled to appear after osteoclasts have finished cutting out a section of bone. The "coupling" process whereby bone resorption leads to bone formation is not understood entirely. The loss of bone with aging results from less bone being formed from osteoblasts than is resorbed by osteoclasts.

In treating osteoporosis, the use of medication to increase bone mass aims at increasing the amount of bone formed by osteoblasts to a level greater than the amount resorbed by osteoclasts. New bone is rapidly formed when the body heals a fracture, and bone cells are responsive even in old age. Understanding the control of bone cells and the coupling process is presently the subject of very intense research and may hold the key to an eventual cure for osteoporosis.

BONES AS ORGANS

There are different types of bones, and each is shaped to perform a specific function. Bones provide strength and shape. They are joined together at joints and are held in the proper position by tendons. Joints allow movement in response to the pull of muscles, and certain ligaments attach muscle to bone whereas others limit the movement of the joints. *Osteoarthritis* is a disorder that affects the joints, whereas osteoporosis is one that affects bone. Osteoarthritis and osteoporosis are unrelated. Some further discussion of the bones that most commonly fracture may be useful. These are the vertebrae, the femur, and the *radius*.

The Spine

The ribs are attached to the *thoracic vertebrae*, which are named according to their positions as D1 (or T1) through D12 (T12) (see Figure 2.4). The thoracic spine curves gently outward. The whole thoracic rib cage moves together so that the thoracic spine receives compression (mechanical force) as a unit.

The section of the spine below the thoracic spine is called the lumbar spine, and the *lumbar vertebrae* are named L1 through L5. The lumbar spine curves in a direction opposite to the thoracic spine.

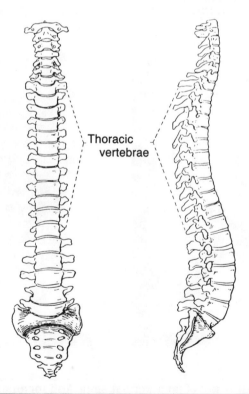

Thoracic
vertebrae

Figure 2.4   The ribs are attached to the thoracic vertebrae, which are named according to their position as D1 (or T1) through D12 (T12).

Lumbar vertebrae are not bolstered by ribs and therefore receive compressive forces individually rather than as a unit. The sacrum is below the lumbar spine and serves as a solid base, being attached both to the lumbar spine and the pelvis.

The vertebral bodies consist of a shell of cortical bone and an inner structure of trabecular bone. Compressive forces to the spine are dissipated by cortical bone and then distributed evenly through the vertebral body by the *trabeculae*, which are struts of trabecular bone that are organized to withstand stress on the spine. Vertical trabeculae withstand the forces on the spine and are reinforced by horizontal trabeculae which act as cross-braces. *Intervertebral disks* are cushionlike structures between vertebrae that function like shock absorbers. The back (posterior) side of a vertebral body is much more stable than the front (anterior) side because the vertebral body's posterior continuation is the *neural arch*, which is supported by spinal muscles and ligaments.

Vertebral fractures are not like breaks in the long bones of the arms and legs. Because the force of gravity on the spine is a vertical force, vertebral fractures result in actual collapses of bone. This means that vertebrae are "crushed" instead of broken apart.

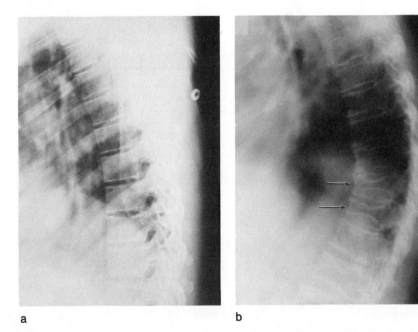

a   b

Figure 2.5 An X ray of (a) a normal spine and (b) an osteoporotic spine. The bone is less dense and wedge and crush fractures are present.

Some parts of the spine are more vulnerable than others to normal compressive forces. The front part of the vertebral body can be compressed more than the back because it does not have the support of the neural arch. This is a *wedge fracture*. When the vertebra becomes too weak, both the front and the back will be compressed. This is a *crush fracture*. Compressive forces are concentrated in two areas: the area of the peak curve of the dorsal spine and the junction of the thoracic and lumbar spines *(thoracolumbar junction)*.

The body's center of gravity is in front of the spine, so the peak curve in the thoracic spine is subject to the greatest force. The thoracic spine acts as a unit and thus places the weight of all its vertebrae on the lumbar spine, often causing compression in the lower thoracic and upper lumbar vertebrae (around the thoracolumbar junction). Compression fractures are common in D6, D10, D11, and D12 and L1 through L3 (Figure 2.5).

The Radius

The radius (wrist) is one of two bones that constitute the forearm. The other bone is the *ulna*, which lies parallel to the radius. The

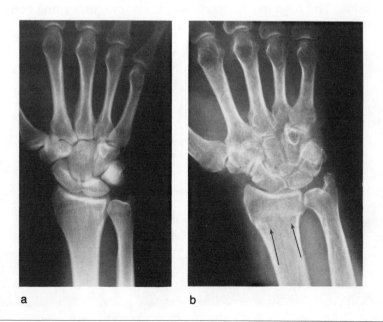

a b

Figure 2.6 An X ray of (a) a normal radius and (b) a radius with a Colles' fractures (indicated by the arrows).

end of the radius near the elbow is a small knob, but near the other end it enlarges so that almost all the joint surface of the forearm side of the wrist is contributed by the radius. This part of the radius can fracture (see Figure 2.6) when someone breaks a fall by landing on an outstretched hand. The radius may be broken and remain in place or may be displaced in several directions. Colles' fracture bears the name of the surgeon who described the displacement of the radius toward the back of the forearm.

The Femur

The femur is the thighbone and a typical long bone. A fracture of the hip refers to the femur. The top end of the femur is a ball that fits into a socket in the pelvis (the acetabulum), allowing rotary motion in the hip joint. The ball continues in the shape of a cylinder (the neck of the femur) and joins the shaft, which is also cylindrical. The angle between the neck and the shaft of the femur is normally 135 degrees. The shaft of the femur ends at the knee with two prominences called condyles. Two bony knobs may be noted on the femur: the greater (larger) trochanter and the lesser trochanter. They are formed by the pulling of the powerful hip muscles. The greater trochanter is on the outside and the lesser on the inside. The intertrochanteric line is an imaginary line connecting the two trochanters (see Figure 2.7).

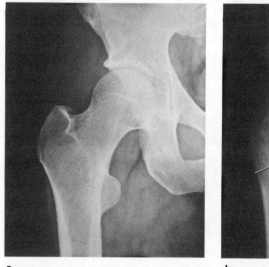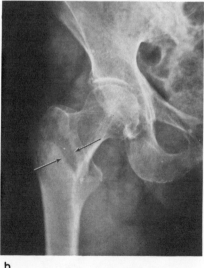

a   b

Figure 2.7 An X ray of (a) a normal femur and (b) a fractured femur (indicated by the arrows).

Unusual forces on the femur result in two sites for osteoporotic fractures: the neck of the femur and along the intertrochanteric line (intertrochanteric fractures).

BONE GAIN AND BONE LOSS

Now that we have considered the skeletal system at its various levels of organization (cells, tissue, and organs), let us consider the changes in skeletal mass that occur in the various stages of the human life cycle. In this section, the gain and loss of bone from the skeleton as a whole will be discussed, followed by a description of how low bone mass may develop. Finally, a distinction will be made between the loss of bone from the skeleton as a whole and the loss from the particular bones that are most subject to osteoporotic fractures.

Women begin life with a lower bone mass than do men. This is one reason why women are more likely to develop osteoporosis. During the first year of life, the skeleton increases more in relation to body size than at any other time in the life cycle (see Figure 2.8 on page 20). During childhood, the skeleton increases in mass with the rest of the body.

Under the influence of the *gonadal hormones* (estrogen in women and testosterone in men), there is a rapid phase of skeletal growth during adolescence. About 45% of adult skeletal mass is formed during adolescence. The skeleton during this rapid phase of growth is not architecturally mature. As a result, during young adulthood (childbearing age in women) the skeleton fills out, and maximal skeletal mass and strength are developed. Thus, bone mass reaches its peak after linear growth (height) has ceased. Indeed, a woman may gain 10% to 15% of her skeletal mass in the reproductive stage of her life cycle. This amount of bone is almost equivalent to the amount lost after menopause. Peak bone mass—the amount of bone present before the onset of bone loss due to aging—is a major determinant of bone mass in later life.

It appears that the highest peak bone mass that can be attained is inherited. However, bone mass can be increased by the mechanical stress put on the skeleton during exercise. Drinking milk in childhood is associated with a higher peak bone mass. Gonadal, or sex, hormones also play a role in achieving maximal peak bone mass. Studies of women who have taken oral contraceptives, which have a very high estrogen content, suggest that they may be protected against osteoporosis in later life.

Around the ages of 35 to 40, a slow loss of bone mass begins in both men and women. Less than .5% is lost from the entire skeleton

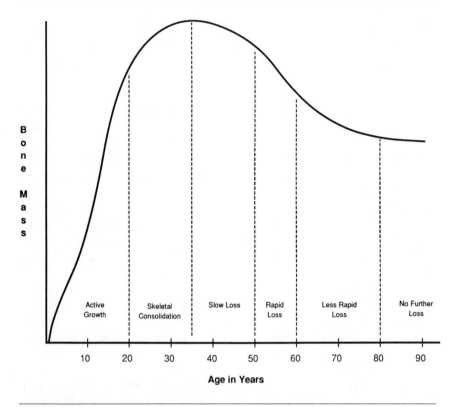

B
o
n
e

M
a
s
s

Active Growth	Skeletal Consolidation	Slow Loss	Rapid Loss	Less Rapid Loss	No Further Loss

10   20   30   40   50   60   70   80   90

Age in Years

Figure 2.8   Stages of bone mass in the life cycle of a woman. Following completion of growth there is another phase of an increase in bone mass at the end of which peak bone mass is attained. This is followed by a slow rate of loss that accelerates following menopause.

annually. This is thought to be due to the aging process or to less stress being exerted on the skeleton as a result of a decrease in physical activity.

Superimposed on this slower rate of bone loss, women experience a rapid rate of loss beginning at menopause. This continues for 5 to 10 years and then reverts to the earlier, slow loss so that, by age 70, women again lose bone mass at the same slow rate that men do.

The Routes to Osteoporosis

Osteoporosis results from developing such a low bone mass that there is a high risk for fracture from minimal mechanical stress. The *fracture threshold* is a theoretical concept that relates the level of bone mass to the risk for fracture. Most women with osteoporotic fractures will have bone-mass measurements below this value. There are many reasons some individuals have lower bone-mass levels in later life. Routes to osteoporosis can be understood by studying Figure 2.9.

The average loss of bone is depicted by line a. Most women will have lost sufficient bone mass by age 80 to be below the fracture threshold and at risk for fracture. Some women will reach adult-hood with a low peak bone mass (line b). As a result, any woman in this category may be below the fracture threshold by age 65 instead of 80. For a woman who has her ovaries removed surgically

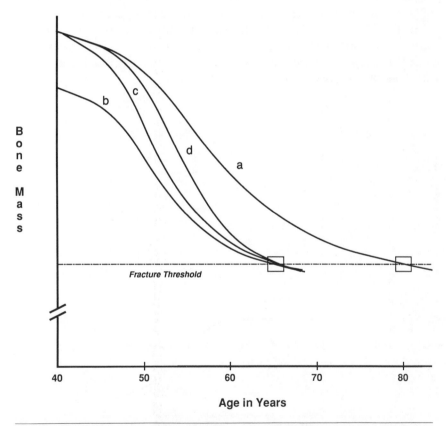

Figure 2.9 Routes to osteoporosis. In the individual with an average peak bone mass, an average rate of bone loss and an average age of menopause (line a), osteoporosis may develop by age 80 years. In the other examples osteoporosis develops earlier because of low peak bone mass (line b), an early menopause (line c), or a more rapid rate of post-menopausal bone loss (line d).

or who has a natural early menopause, the rapid loss of bone that ordinarily occurs around age 50 starts earlier so that, at age 65, bone mass is below the fracture threshold (line c). Finally, some women have more rapid bone loss than others and will be below the fracture level even though they have average peak bone mass (line d). So those at high risk for osteoporosis are mainly women with low peak bone mass, an early menopause, or a more rapid than average loss of bone mass after menopause.

Bone Loss From the Radius, Spine, and Femur

The patterns of bone loss I have discussed so far describe what happens to the skeleton as a whole. The entire skeleton is composed of 80% cortical bone; the spine and femur have a greater proportion of trabecular bone. Recent studies have shown that a substantial amount of bone is lost from the spine and femur prior to menopause. It seems likely that the loss of trabecular bone begins earlier than the loss of cortical bone (see Figure 2.10).

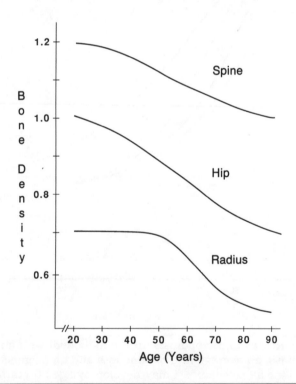

Figure 2.10 Loss of bone density with age. Note that bone loss begins before menopause from the spine and hip whereas the greatest amount of bone is lost from the radius after menopause.

If osteoporosis is to be prevented, attention must be focused on the factors that influence bone mass in each stage of the life cycle. The development of maximal bone mass by early adulthood is as important as preventing bone loss in later life.

OSTEOPOROSIS CLASSIFICATION

Now that you better understand calcium homeostasis and the skeletal system, the classification of osteoporosis will be discussed. Osteoporosis may be classified as a primary or secondary disease. *Primary osteoporosis* is diagnosed only after excluding all possibilities of a link to another illness. *Secondary osteoporosis* is diagnosed when the condition is linked to another illness such as kidney disease or to prolonged medical treatment involving the use of certain medications. Table 2.1 lists other factors that can contribute to secondary osteoporosis.

Age groups are also used to classify osteoporosis. *Juvenile osteoporosis* affects prepubescent boys and girls. *Idiopathic osteoporosis*

Table 2.1   Factors Contributing to Secondary Osteoporosis

Drugs	Endocrine
Glucocorticoids	Hypogonadism
Heparin	Cushing's syndrome
Anticonvulsants	Hyperparathyroidism
Alcohol	Hyperthyroidism
Methotrexate	Growth hormone deficiency
Congenital Conditions	**Others**
Osteogenesis imperfecta	Renal tubular acidosis
Hypophosphatasia	Rheumatoid arthritis
Homocystinuria	Immobilization
Hemolytic anemia	Mastocytosis
Diet	Liver disease
Malabsorption syndromes	Multiple myeloma, lymphoma
Calcium deficiency	Leukemia
Starvation	
Scurvy	

describes the condition in young adults of either sex when the cause is unknown. *Postmenopausal osteoporosis* occurs in women within 15 to 20 years after menopause. *Senile or involutional osteoporosis* is used primarily to describe the disease in the elderly.

Recently, researchers at the Mayo Clinic (Riggs et al., 1982b) have suggested that osteoporosis be classified as *Type I* and *Type II*. Type I is equivalent to postmenopausal osteoporosis and Type II to involutional osteoporosis. Type I affects women within 15 to 20 years after menopause and is associated with crush fractures of the spine and fractures of the wrist. Type II affects men and women over age 70 and is associated with wedge fractures of the spine and fractures of the hip.

The Mayo researchers have proposed that the two types of osteoporosis may have different causes. Type I is believed to occur in a small group of women who have an unusually great loss of trabecular bone and are therefore prone to vertebral crush fractures or Colles' fracture (if they happen to fall). The major cause of this type of osteoporosis is postmenopausal bone loss, although low peak bone mass may also play a role. The Mayo group proposes that the loss of bone that occurs with aging is the cause of Type II, in which there is proportionate loss of cortical and trabecular bone from the spine and femur as a result of aging. By age 80, there is sufficient loss of cortical and trabecular bone of the femur to place most individuals at risk for hip fracture. The loss of bone due to aging

Table 2.2   Factors Influencing Postmenopausal (Type I) and Involutional (Type II) Osteoporosis

Factors	Type I	Type II
Age	55 to 75	> 70
Sex (F:M)	6:1	2:1
Fracture types	Wrist/vertebrae	Hip/vertebrae, long bones
Hormonal cause	Estrogen deficiency	Calcitriol deficiency
Calcium absorption	Decreased	Decreased
Increased parathyroid hormone	No	Yes
Importance of dietary calcium	Moderate	High

may also result in the gradual deformation of the spine in the form of wedge fractures (see Table 2.2).

Let us review why parathyroid hormone is considered central to the development of both Type I and Type II osteoporosis. Remember that calcium (skeletal) balance becomes slightly negative in the third decade of life. Many scientists believe that this is an effect of reduced physical activity, resulting in osteoblasts only partially filling resorption cavities with new bone.

The magnitude of bone loss with aging is determined by the number of active remodeling units. If the calcium balance is slightly negative at each remodeling unit and the number of units is increased dramatically, there will be a significant loss of skeletal mass. Parathyroid hormone normally increases the number of remodeling units. Therefore, an increase in the amount or effectiveness of parathyroid hormone will result in greater bone loss. Conversely, a reduction in the amount or effectiveness of parathyroid hormone will result in less bone loss.

Some recent and fascinating studies may partially explain the finding that blacks have a higher bone mass than whites (Bell et al., 1985). The skeleton of some black Americans is resistant to parathyroid hormone; that is, the effectiveness of parathyroid hormone is diminished. Calcium resorption from bone is thus reduced, and blood levels of calcium fall. The decline of blood calcium levels is a stimulus for release of yet more parathyroid hormone. The increase in parathyroid hormone results in increased absorption of calcium at the kidneys. Thus, the blood levels are preserved without incurring calcium loss in the bone.

Because estrogens antagonize the effect of parathyroid hormone, estrogen deficiency following menopause results in an increase in the sensitivity of bone to parathyroid hormone. More remodeling units result in greater loss of bone mass and contribute to the development of Type I osteoporosis. In contrast, the reduction of the kidney's ability to manufacture calcitriol (vitamin D) results in Type II osteoporosis. Type II osteoporosis is thus characterized by reduced calcium absorption, which in turn results in increased secretion of parathyroid hormone. Once again, the number of remodeling units increases and bone mass is lost.

SUMMARY

The skeleton changes shape by forming new bone in response to mechanical stress. This process is called modeling. The skeleton is continuously being remodeled: Osteoclasts first dissolve bone, then osteoblasts lay down the soft bone matrix and osteocytes initiate the process of depositing mineral crystals in the matrix.

The two types of skeletal tissue are cortical bone and trabecular bone. The sites of the skeleton that are subject to osteoporotic fractures normally have a greater amount of trabecular bone. Osteoporosis is a metabolic bone disease in which bone composition is normal. Osteomalacia is an example of a bone disease in which composition is not normal; an increased amount of unmineralized matrix develops.

The vertebrae, the radius, and the femur are the bones that commonly fracture in women with osteoporosis. The vertical forces to which the spine is exposed compress the vertebrae, resulting in compression fractures, which are further classified as wedge and crush fractures. Colles' fracture occurs in the radius. The femur can fracture either in the neck or along the intertrochanteric line.

Females begin life with a lower bone mass than males. Both sexes experience a great increase in skeletal mass during childhood; about 45% of adult skeletal mass is formed during adolescence, followed by a further increase of 10% to 15% during young adulthood. Peak bone mass is a major determinant of bone mass in later life. Women begin to lose bone around the age of 35 to 40; this process accelerates after menopause and then resumes at the slower rate of loss. This model describes body loss from the entire skeleton, but substantial loss of trabecular bone also occurs before menopause. This means that the loss of bone from the femur and vertebrae precedes the loss from the whole body or the radius.

Researchers classify osteoporosis as either primary or secondary to another disease. Primary osteoporosis is subclassified as juvenile, idiopathic, postmenopausal (Type I), and involutional (Type II). Type I osteoporosis results from postmenopausal bone loss and is associated with crush fractures of the vertebrae and Colles' fractures. Type II osteoporosis occurs in older individuals and is associated with wedge fractures of the spine and fractures of the hip.

3 CHAPTER

Osteoporosis Risk Factors

The adage "An ounce of prevention is worth a pound of cure" has special relevance to osteoporosis. Can you prevent fractures that occur with postmenopausal osteoporosis? The answer is a resounding "Yes!" Prevention begins by adopting and maintaining a healthy lifestyle, identifying and reducing risk factors in menopausal women, and minimizing the elderly's risk of falling and injuring the spine.

MODIFIABLE AND NONMODIFIABLE RISK FACTORS

Only recently have we begun to think of osteoporosis in the same way that we think of *atherosclerosis* (hardening of the arteries). We all lose bone mass as we age, but we may be able to minimize this loss by reducing both individual and environmental risk factors. We can't do anything about some risk factors for osteoporosis, such as the presence of *scoliosis* (which is inherited), whereas we can reduce or modify others, such as a low-calcium diet.

The following risk factors for osteoporosis can't be influenced by diet, activity, or medication:

- Being a Caucasian or Asian female
- Having a family history of the disease
- Having light skin
- Having a small frame
- Experiencing previous bone loss due to immobilization, hyperparathyroidism, thyrotoxicosis, liver disease, malabsorption, rheumatoid arthritis, chronic illness, or glucocorticoids and other drugs
- Having scoliosis
- Suffering previous osteoporotic fractures

The following risk factors can be influenced by diet, activity, and medication:

- Estrogen deficiency (early menopause, oophorectomy)
- Inactivity
- Low-calcium diet
- Cigarette smoking
- Excess consumption of protein, caffeine, alcohol, and phosphorus
- Vitamin D deficiency or altered metabolism of vitamin D
- Low weight relative to height

Osteoporosis is usually a silent illness, like a heart attack. In some people coronary arteries begin to narrow before age 30, so that by the time they reach 55, their blood vessels are so narrow that they suffer a heart attack. Similarly, the steady reduction of a woman's bone mass is silent and eventually results in a critically low bone mass that leaves her subject to catastrophic fractures, such as those of the vertebra.

Of course, not everyone suffers a heart attack or an osteoporotic fracture under these conditions. Some people are at a higher risk for these events due to risk factors. Multiple risk factors for heart attack include heredity, sex, race, age, blood cholesterol level, and hypertension (high blood pressure). As you will see in this chapter, osteoporosis and atherosclerosis are similar in that they both involve multiple risk factors.

The various kinds of osteoporotic fractures share common risk factors because the same factors influence bone mass and strength in the wrist, hip, and spine. The major difference between women with vertebral fractures and women of the same age without fractures is the density of their spines. In contrast, hip-fracture patients also have osteoporosis, but, when compared with individuals of the same age without fractures, less difference exists between the two in bone mass. The difference between these two groups is that the individuals with hip fractures fell.

This chapter discusses bone mass and strength and recommends ways to maximize bone mass. Chapter 4 describes ways to minimize mechanical stress on the skeleton.

THE INFLUENCE OF HEREDITY ON PEAK BONE MASS

The peak bone mass that any individual can attain is probably genetically determined. Men have a higher bone mass than do women throughout life. Twins have similar bone mass. A small bone frame is inherited. Although there is little information concerning whether rates of bone loss are also under genetic influence, it is known that, if your mother had osteoporosis, you are more likely to develop it. Black Americans, both men and women, have a higher bone mass than whites have. As a result, osteoporosis is an unusual disorder in blacks. It is evident, however, that osteoporosis is a worldwide problem. It occurs in those of yellow and brown skin as well as in the classic osteoporotic stereotype of a slender, fair-skinned woman of northern European origin.

THE EFFECTS OF INACTIVITY AND ACTIVITY ON BONE MASS

Immobilization (bed rest) causes rapid bone loss. This was noticed many years ago when patients with fractures were immobilized in whole-body casts. The patients lost bone very rapidly and excreted a large amount of calcium in their urine. Studies on these patients revealed that the negative calcium balance could be corrected only by bearing weight. Exercise that did not involve weight bearing did not protect against bone loss.

A similar problem has arisen in space travel. One of the limitations of space travel is that weightlessness results in rapid bone loss. There have been a number of studies performed on U.S. space flights and some on Soviet space flights as well to determine how to prevent bone loss. These attempts have met with little success, and it may be that this consequence of weightlessness will be a limitation to prolonged space flight.

On the other hand, exercise increases bone mass. The mass of a muscle in an arm, for example, is proportional to the mass of bone in the same extremity. Evidence of localized *hypertrophy* (increase in mass) of bone has been gained from studies of athletes (Nilsson & Westlin, 1971). Tennis players have a high density of bone in their playing arms. The same has been found for lumberjacks and baseball players (Aloia, 1981). Winthrop/Brookhaven researchers studied male marathon runners and found that their total skeletal mass did not decrease with age (Aloia, Cohn, Babu, et al., 1978).

It has been difficult to demonstrate a relationship between physical activity and bone mass in *sedentary* populations because it is difficult to measure physical activity accurately. This problem has been overcome recently by the use of a sensor that determines the amount of body motion. One study (Black-Sandler et al., 1982) showed that the bone mass of the forearm is related to exercise as detected by a motion sensor. This was the case in a sedentary post-menopausal population of women. Using motion sensors, the Brook-haven/Winthrop research group (Aloia, Vaswani, Yeh, & Cohn, 1988) observed a relationship between bone mass and activity in sedentary premenopausal women, indicating that even a little exercise may be beneficial.

Several other studies have also shown that bone loss in post-menopausal women may be prevented by exercise. The Brookhaven/Winthrop research group (Aloia, Cohn, Ostuni, Cane, & Ellis, 1978) enrolled a group of volunteer women in an exercise program and compared them to a group that did not exercise. The exercises used were suggested by the President's Council on Physical Fitness. After 2 years, there was no loss of bone in the exercise group, whereas the expected loss occurred in the control (nonexercise) group. It has been shown in an elderly population that physical exercise retards bone loss (Smith, Reddan, & Smith, 1981).

The evidence supporting the positive effect of physical activity on maintaining or increasing bone mass is quite strong. Recent research suggests that mechanical forces influence osteoblasts to form new bone. Many researchers believe that the slow loss of bone in aging men and women is due to a reduction in osteoblastic function, which could be due to physical inactivity. It is important to realize that skeletal mass adapts to the mechanical load placed on the skeleton. If years of high physical activity are followed by years of inactivity the bone that was gained earlier will be lost.

THE EFFECTS OF NUTRITION ON BONE MASS

A number of dietary factors have been implicated in the development of osteoporosis. Excess phosphorus in the diet may cause bone loss. The studies that were performed to demonstrate this involved high amounts of dietary phosphorus, much higher than the amounts generally eaten by the average American. However, some individuals do drink a large amount of carbonated soft drinks, which contain approximately 20 milligrams per 100 milliliters of phosphorus. It is certainly conceivable that an individual who is drinking six cans of soda per day could experience some bone loss. Caffeine and excess alcohol may also produce bone loss. Their consumption should be limited.

Adolescents and Low Calorie Diets

Frequent starvation diets will lower bone mass. This has become a great concern because of the increasing number both of adolescent girls who are dieting and of patients with *anorexia nervosa*. Very low calorie diets increase urinary loss of calcium and lead to bone loss. High-protein diets also increase urinary calcium loss. The recommended dietary protein content for optimal nutrition is 20% of total calories.

Calcium intake is important in maintaining bone mass as well as in developing maximal peak bone mass. Prior to the current media attention to preventing osteoporosis through calcium supplementation, many American women had a low dietary calcium intake. Calcium intake and other aspects of nutrition will be discussed in detail in chapters 5 and 6.

The Elderly and Vitamin D

The elderly often have both a reduced dietary intake of vitamin D and a reduced exposure to sunlight. Osteoporotic women may manufacture less vitamin D in their skin following exposure to sunlight. Remember that the elderly have a reduced ability to manufacture calcitriol (the active form of vitamin D) and therefore have a reduced ability to absorb calcium from their diets. Theoretically, this could be overcome by providing large amounts of calcium supplements or by taking vitamin D or calcitriol. It seems wise to provide supplements of 400 international units (IU) of vitamin D per day to the elderly, particularly if they are homebound or have a low level of vitamin D in the blood. However, physicians must be cautious when prescribing larger amounts of vitamin D as taking excessive amounts of this vitamin can produce high levels of blood and urine calcium as well as kidney stones. In addition, high levels of vitamin D probably produce bone loss rather than gain.

ESTROGEN'S EFFECT ON BONE MASS

As a result of the loss of estrogen following menopause there is an increase in bone resorption (bone loss) and a decrease in the ability to absorb calcium from the diet. A woman who has had her ovaries removed surgically or who has an early menopause undergoes a similar rapid phase of bone loss. An early menopause is a powerful risk factor for osteoporosis. Indeed, the number of years of estrogen deficiency is more important than a woman's age in influencing the extent of bone loss she has experienced. If you need a *hysterectomy*, consider the possibility of leaving your ovaries intact.

Although some studies suggest that estrogen needs to be given within the first 3 to 6 years following the surgical removal of the ovaries *(oophorectomy)*, other studies have shown that there is a benefit even at a later age. However, estrogen-replacement therapy should be thought of as a way to prevent further bone loss rather than as a way to produce a marked increase in bone mass. If one stops bone loss at age 40, the effect will be different from that if estrogens were started at age 60. At the later age, the individual may have lost about 20% of skeletal mass. Thus, estrogen-replacement therapy at age 60 would leave the patient with a deficit of at least 20% in skeletal mass. This is a level that will leave the patient at high risk for the development of osteoporotic fractures (see Figure 3.1).

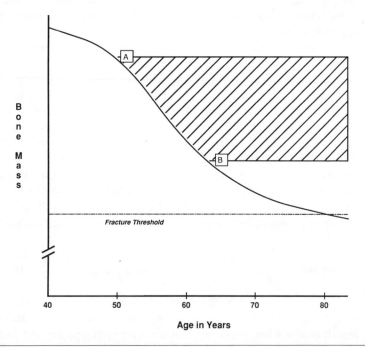

Figure 3.1   The varied influence of beginning estrogen treatment at different times after the menopause. Bone loss ceases in both example A and B. However, there is less benefit when estrogen is given at age 65 rather than at menopause because of the amount of bone mass that was lost prior to treatment.

Another important concept involves the relative merits of exercise and estrogen. Women who exercise to the extreme of developing amenorrhea (cessation of periods associated with, in this case, estrogen deficiency) lose bone more rapidly than normal. The condition of exercise-induced amenorrhea is associated with osteoporosis. Therefore, adequate exercise is important, but adequate estrogen levels are even more important. Exercise in premenopausal women that is so extreme that it results in menstrual irregularity or amenorrhea is not helpful in preventing osteoporosis. It is essential to adequately increase dietary intake when embarking on a strenuous exercise program so that estrogen deficiency may be prevented.

A study of ballet dancers conducted by Columbia University researchers (Warren, Brooks-Gunn, Hamilton, Warren, & Hamilton, 1986) may provide the connection between scoliosis and osteoporosis. The Columbia investigators found that one quarter of the ballet dancers had scoliosis. The dancers with scoliosis had more evidence of estrogen deficiency and dieted more severely. They frequently started having periods later (delayed menarche) or had amenorrhea. Stress fractures were more common in the dancers with delayed menarche or amenorrhea. Thus, scoliosis may be indirectly related to osteoporosis, with both illnesses resulting from a common cause, that is, estrogen deficiency.

OTHER HORMONES' EFFECTS ON BONE MASS

The roles of parathyroid hormone and calcitriol in the development of osteoporosis were discussed in chapter 2. Blood levels of calcitonin are lower in women than in men and decline with aging. Therefore, calcitonin deficiency may hasten the development of osteoporosis.

Cortisol, the most important hormone made by the adrenal glands, has also been implicated in bone loss. Some researchers believe that a relative excess of cortisol with a deficiency of calcitonin, secondary to a lack of estrogen, results in osteoporosis. There is less evidence that other hormones are implicated in the case of osteoporosis. Thus, testosterone levels may decline in older age, resulting in decreased bone mass in men and women. Growth hormone also decreases with aging, and some studies suggest that growth hormone may play a role in the development of osteoporosis. However, of all the possible hormonal mechanisms, it is clear that estrogen withdrawal at the time of menopause is the most important cause of accelerated bone loss in women. Calcitriol deficiency and inactivity may be more important in the elderly.

CIGARETTE SMOKING'S EFFECTS ON BONE MASS

Cigarette smoking is another cause of low bone mass and osteoporosis. It may be difficult to believe that cigarettes could be harmful for everything—the heart, the lungs, and even the bones! However, comparison of osteoporotic patients with age-matched controls at Brookhaven National Laboratory revealed a higher incidence of cigarette smoking in osteoporotic patients (Aloia et al., 1985). In another study it was observed that women who smoke increase their risk of hip fracture 1.7 times. In women, 10% to 20% of hip fractures are attributable to smoking.

Women who smoke undergo an early menopause. This may result in a longer period of estrogen deficiency and, therefore, a longer period of bone loss. Cigarettes may also reduce calcium absorption. Recent studies by Danish researchers (Jensen, Christiansen, & Rodbro, 1985) show that cigarette smoking affects estrogen metabolism. Women who take estrogens have lower blood levels of estrogen if they smoke.

THE EFFECTS OF DRUGS AND ILLNESSES ON BONE MASS

A variety of drugs are known to cause bone loss. The use of cortisol (glucocorticoid drugs) is associated with the rapid development of osteoporosis. These drugs are primarily used to treat patients with asthma and rheumatic disorders. A number of other medications have also been associated with the development of osteoporosis. *Hyperthyroidism* (an overactive thyroid gland) can produce bone loss, as can taking an excess amount of thyroid hormone. Individuals taking thyroid hormone replacement therapy are at a greater risk for developing osteoporosis. If you take thyroid hormone, have your physician check whether the dose is excessive. This can be done with a blood test called a Thyroid Stimulating Hormone level. Certain *diuretics* (water pills) such as furosemide cause an increase in calcium excretion. The prolonged use of aluminum-containing antacids has been implicated in bone loss. These antacids include Amphojel, Maalox, Gelusil, Aludrox, and Mylanta. The regular use of these antacids may increase calcium requirements by as much as 500 mg per day. Anticonvulsant medication interferes with vitamin D metabolism and may cause bone loss. All these drugs should be avoided if possible, but if it is necessary to take them, consider supplementing your diet with calcium and vitamin D.

A list of drugs that may produce bone loss follows:

- Glucocorticoids
- Thyroid hormone in excess
- Antiestrogens
- Gonadotropin-releasing hormone agonist (for endometriosis)
- Antacids containing aluminum
- Loop diuretics
- Tetracycline
- Isoniazide
- Anticonvulsants

Any illness that results in poor nutrition or prolonged bed rest can produce bone loss. The illnesses classified under secondary osteoporosis in Table 2.1 are especially important. Calcium absorption is decreased by gastric surgery, diseases of the small intestine, liver disease, and kidney failure. Calcitriol is used in the treatment of individuals with kidney failure to prevent the bone loss that results from the inability of diseased kidneys to manufacture calcitriol.

AN OSTEOPOROSIS RISK QUIZ AND PREVENTION COMMANDMENTS

The osteoporosis risk quiz is designed to help you assess your risk for osteoporosis.

An Osteoporosis Risk Quiz

	Yes	No
1. Are you a white or Asian menopausal woman?	___	___
2. Did your mother or sister have osteoporosis?	___	___
3. Did you have your ovaries removed surgically, have early menopause, or have prolonged amenorrhea?	___	___
4. Did you decide not to take estrogen after menopause?	___	___

(Cont.)

An Osteoporosis Risk Quiz (Continued)

	Yes	No
5. Did you diet frequently?	___	___
6. Do you smoke?	___	___
7. Do you drink excessively?	___	___
8. Has your dietary calcium intake been low?	___	___
9. Were you sedentary as a child or young adult?	___	___
10. Were you ever confined to bed for a long time?	___	___
11. Did you take medication that causes bone loss?	___	___
12. Do you have scoliosis?	___	___
13. Have you had any illness that causes bone loss?	___	___

If you answered yes to one or more of these questions you may be at risk for developing osteoporosis.

After taking this quiz, you may wonder what measures can be recommended for preventing osteoporosis. The ten commandments of prevention reflect the information you have learned about modifiable risk factors.

The Ten Commandments of Osteoporosis Prevention

1. Get enough calcium in a balanced diet.
2. Get enough vitamin D in your diet and from sunshine.
3. Limit your intake of caffeine, salt, protein, and phosphorus.
4. Do not go on starvation diets.
5. Exercise regularly.
6. Take estrogen (progesterone after menopause if you are at high risk for osteoporosis).
7. Take estrogen if your ovaries have been removed surgically before menopause.
8. Avoid drugs that decrease bone mass.
9. Drink alcohol only in moderation.
10. Do not smoke.

Implementing these lifestyle changes may not be easy. Suggestions for doing so will be provided in following chapters.

FACTORS INFLUENCING BONE STRENGTH

Although bone mass is proportional to bone strength, the two cannot always be equated. There are several factors that decrease the strength of bone independently of its mass: (a) reduced material strength, (b) inadequate microfracture repair, and (c) altered bony architecture. Bone may be considered from the viewpoint of an engineer, with the recognition that not only is the mass of material critical but so is its composition and structure. This area of research is very active at present, but little is known about bone strength compared to what is known about bone mass.

REDUCED BONE STRENGTH

The strength of bone is related not only to the amount of mineral but also to the composition and structure of the combined mineral and matrix. Bone may have a normal density and yet be subject to fracture because of increased brittleness or softness. An example of the former is *fluoridic bone* (bone containing excess fluoride), which may even have an increased density and yet fracture more readily because of increased brittleness. Increased softness is a more common occurrence. In Great Britain, some patients with fractured hips have been found to have osteomalacia on bone biopsy (unmineralized osteoid may contribute to fracture). In the United States, a study of patients with fractured hips revealed subclinical, or mild, osteomalacia. These patients did not have obvious osteomalacia (even on bone biopsy), but there was a somewhat increased amount of unmineralized bone matrix. Although severe osteomalacia is uncommon in the United States, this subclinical form of osteomalacia may contribute to the risk for hip fracture in the elderly.

Inadequate Microfracture Repair

Engineers are familiar with metal fatigue or stress cracks that develop in most structural material, including stone and concrete. These minor cracks, unless repaired, can gradually increase in size until the structure has major defects. Then minor mechanical stress may result in structural failure. A similar process occurs in bone. The number of microfractures increases with aging and is highest in areas of the spine that are most susceptible to fracture (L2 through L4). The body's way of repairing microfractures is through bone remodeling. The area with the stress crack is removed by bone resorption and replaced with new bone.

A major theoretical concern with drug treatment for osteoporosis that reduces bone remodeling is that there could be an increase in the number of microfractures, resulting in decreased bone strength even if there were an increase in bone mass. Drug treatment for osteoporosis should demonstrate a reduction in fracture rate to be considered effective.

Altered Bone Architecture

There are two changes in the architecture of bone that may predispose the vertebrae and femur to fracture in osteoporosis. It has recently been shown that there are two patterns of loss of trabecular bone with aging. In women with postmenopausal osteoporosis, cross-bracing trabeculae are lost. In older men, all the trabeculae are intact but simply become thinner. For an equal bone mass, this latter structure is stronger.

In the femur, as in all long bones, the *periosteal* (outer) diameter of the bone expands with age. This reduces the resilience of the shaft of the femur and transfers the area that is most stressed to the proximal femur, the common site for hip fractures.

SUMMARY

The risk for fracture is related to trauma to the skeleton and the skeleton's ability to withstand that trauma. Bone strength is determined primarily by bone mass but also by bone quality, bone architecture, and the adequacy of microfracture repair. Most of the information we have gathered to date has to do with bone mass. Our bone mass in later life is the result of the interaction between peak bone mass in adulthood and subsequent bone loss. A person's peak bone mass is primarily influenced by heredity, nutrition, and exercise. Extreme exercise that is not accompanied by increased calorie intake may result in amenorrhea and reduced bone mass in premenopausal athletes.

The loss of estrogen around menopause results in accelerated bone loss. Supplemental estrogens prevent postmenopausal bone loss, but we don't know yet whether the same is true for increasing calcium intake. Excessive dietary phosphate and protein may promote bone loss, as may caffeine and alcohol consumption, cigarette smoking, and taking certain medications. The elderly often have mild vitamin D deficiencies. Several hormones may also contribute to bone loss through aging.

You can prevent osteoporosis by adopting and maintaining a healthy lifestyle of good nutrition and exercise and avoiding excess alcohol, tobacco, and certain medications. In addition, menopausal women who are at risk for osteoporosis should be given estrogens. In later life, preventing falls becomes essential in avoiding osteoporotic fractures. This last point is discussed in chapter 4.

4 CHAPTER

Avoiding Osteoporotic Injuries

The risk for fracture is related not only to the strength of a particular bone, but also to the stress it must withstand. However, the role of force in causing osteoporotic fractures depends on the location of the fracture. A Colles' fracture, for instance, always results from a person's breaking a fall with an outstretched hand. Individuals under 70 are the most likely to fracture a wrist, primarily as a result of slipping or tripping. In contrast, spinal fractures have nothing to do with falling. Osteoporotic women may suffer a fracture of the spine by bending or lifting incorrectly or simply by carrying the weight of the body.

Hip fractures can also occur from carrying the weight of the body. A stress fracture progresses to a full fracture over several days—in such cases, we say the person "fractured first and then fell." However, over 80% of individuals with hip fractures actually "fell first and then fractured."

Women who have suffered spinal fractures are distinguished from women of the same age without fractures by the low bone-mineral density of their spines. However, most elderly individuals have a low bone-mineral density of the hip regardless of whether they have suffered a fracture. The 80-year-old woman who broke her hip today had the same bone strength yesterday. The difference is that she fell today. One study (Brocklehurst, Exton-Smith, Lempert-Barber, Hunt, & Palmer, 1978) identified the reasons for falling in most individuals as tripping or slipping (50%), loss of balance (20%), *drop attack* (suddenly falling to the ground) or *syncope* (loss of consciousness) (20%), and miscellaneous (10%).

Developing and maintaining maximal bone strength is the best way to prevent osteoporotic fractures (see Figure 4.1). However, avoiding injury is critical for individuals who already have reduced bone strength.

An individual can minimize the impact of forces on a weakened spine by practicing proper posture and correct lifting and bending techniques. Preventing falls is the major way to avoid fractures of the femur. In addition, you can reduce the impact of a fall by learning protective responses and by strengthening the muscles around the hip that absorb some of the force of impact.

This chapter helps those individuals who have osteoporosis avoid injury by looking at falling and tripping in detail and then outlining ways to avoid spinal injury through proper posture and correct weight-bearing techniques. The chapter ends with a lifelong strategy for preventing osteoporotic fractures by optimizing bone strength and avoiding injury.

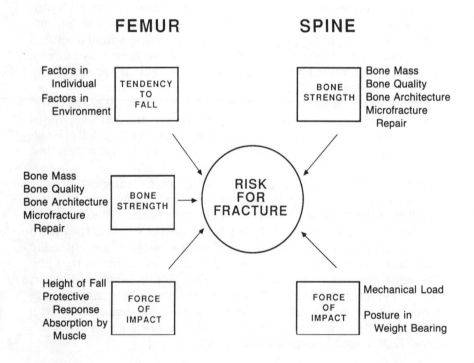

Figure 4.1   Many factors influence the risk of fracture of the spine and femur.

RISKS FOR TRIPPING AND FALLING IN THE ELDERLY

Accidents are the fifth-highest cause of death in later life. Seventy-five percent of accidental deaths are associated with falls. The Public Health Service estimates that there are 13.6 million falls in the United States per year. Falls are more common in the elderly, in females, and in those who are not living with a spouse. A group of researchers observed that one third of people over 65 fall once or more a year (Campbell, Reinken, Allan, & Martinez, 1981). In another study of 2,793 respondents 65 and older, 28% fell in the past year (Gryfe, Amies, & Ashley, 1977). The rate increased with aging and was twice as high in women as in men. It is evident that the likelihood of falling is alarmingly high in elderly individuals.

Most falls occur from underfoot accidents (tripping). Factors that make the elderly more prone to tripping and falling are displayed in the boxed area.

Reasons the Elderly Are Prone to Tripping and Falling

- Decreased height of stepping (tripping)
- Loss of postural control, or increased sway
- Slowed decision making
- Decreased alertness
- Decreased responsiveness
- Reduced peripheral proprioception
- Decreased vision
- Decreased hearing
- *Postural hypotension*
- Decreased muscle strength and tone
- Illness
- *Arthritis*
- Neurologic disability (stroke, Parkinson's disease)
- Cerebrovascular insufficiency
- Cardiac rhythm disturbance
- Drop attacks
- *Vertigo*

In most surveys it is noted that the young and the old fall frequently. In the young, environmental factors are more important, whereas factors present in the individual predominate in the elderly.

The Causes of Tripping

A large number of the falls due to tripping occur in the bedroom at night and on the stairs. The elderly are more likely to sustain injuries from tripping for a variety of reasons:

- The elderly, once they stumble, cannot correct their balance as rapidly as can the young. Athletes escape injury by knowing how to break the impact of a fall. The elderly individual, however, with slowed reaction time and weak muscles, may not be able to break a fall. An impaired sense of balance makes dependence on visual cues important for the elderly.
- Gait changes with aging. Men bend forward slightly, and their arms and knees are flexed. There is less arm swing and shorter step length. The feet are not raised off the floor as much. Elderly women have a shortened step length and more narrow-based gait that resembles a waddle. As one grows older, there is reduced movement at the pelvis, leading to the inability to raise the feet appropriately. When walking, the pelvis is displaced toward the weight-bearing leg so that the other leg can swing forward. Because the pelvis does not shift adequately, the foot swings too low, resulting in a trip.
- Studies of the ability to perceive whether a rod is vertical or horizontal have shown that visual perception declines with aging (Tobis, Nayak, & Hoehler, 1981). Moreover, visual perception is impaired in those who fall when compared to age-matched normals.
- In addition to reduced perception of objects in the environment, there may be reduced alertness in the elderly. There is a slowing of the decision-making process, and less attention is paid to maintaining balance. Certain drugs may also reduce alertness (Overstall, 1980).

The Causes of Falling

Almost half the falls in the elderly are due to accidents (or tripping). In the other half, the patient suddenly falls to the ground. The most common problems causing sudden falls are drop attacks and postural hypotension. Let us first review the changes in postural sway that occur with aging.

When you stand quietly with your feet together and eyes closed, you will sway back and forth to a slight degree. *Proprioceptive signals* are carried to the brain so that balance is maintained. Children have more positional sway and reach optimal control in the late teens. This remains optimal until about age 60, when there is a progressive increase in sway. The amount of sway can be measured with an instrument called an *ataxiameter*. Sway is greater in women at all ages.

Tripping is not related to sway. Sway is increased in both men and women who fall because of impaired balance. It is increased in women who fall because of giddiness, drop attacks, turning the head, and rising from a bed or chair. This decline in postural control with aging may be accentuated by brain disease (Overstall, Exton-Smith, Imms, & Johnson, 1977).

Drop attacks describe episodes in which an individual suddenly falls to the floor and are due to a reduced blood flow to the brain stem, which is the area of the brain that contains the posture centers. There are a variety of causes of drop attacks, including abnormal cardiac rhythms and *cerebrovascular insufficiency*. Those who suffer these attacks should have a thorough evaluation of their heart and cerebral circulation. The cardiac study that is usually required is a *Holter monitor*. This small instrument records the cardiac rhythm over a 24-hour period. A test that uses ultrasound *(Doppler)* can measure blood flow to the brain.

When you stand, the blood in the circulatory system is pooled in the legs. As a result, less blood is returned to the heart, and blood pressure drops. Less blood will be pumped to the brain, and unconsciousness may follow. In a normal individual, the nervous system compensates for the pooling of blood. *Baroreceptors* (pressure detectors) in the heart and blood vessels detect whether blood pressure is adequate. When these receptors detect low pressure, they signal the brain to activate the sympathetic nervous system. Hormones *(catecholamines)* are secreted from nerve endings that act on blood vessels to restore blood volume and pressure. When this response to standing is impaired, postural hypotension occurs. On assuming an upright position, an individual with postural hypotension may suffer a drop in blood pressure in excess of 20 to 30 mm Hg. Postural hypotension may occur simply with age and is associated with increased sway. *Psychotropic* and *antihypertensive drugs* also cause postural hypotension.

There are a number of reasons women fall more frequently than do men. Drop attacks are more common in women. Women may be more dependent than men are on visual spatial information; those women who fall frequently tend to have impaired vision. More women than men take psychotropic drugs. Also, women have greater postural sway. For all these reasons (as well as their lower bone mass), it is important for women to take measures to avoid falls.

HOW TO AVOID
TRIPPING AND FALLING

Many accidents occur in the bathroom and kitchen. Go through your home with a friend or relative with the objective of finding ways to avoid fracture. Make a list of things you do by habit that may be dangerous; have a personal list of "don'ts." Listen to your friend or relative who counsels you about dangerous activities. One of your don'ts should be *"Don't be stubborn."* The health behavior tips listed in the shaded boxed area provide more information about avoiding falls.

Health Behavior Tips to Avoid Falls

- Go for regular checkups.
- Maintain confidence.
- Have vision checked and corrected.
- Exercise regularly.
- Do postural exercises.
- Rise slowly; don't rush to answer the telephone.
- Avoid hazardous conditions.
- Don't hurry.
- Don't drink alcohol excessively.
- Discuss drugs with your physician.
- Have thorough medical investigation for cause of falls.
- Have hearing checked and corrected.
- Learn to use adaptive devices properly (cane, crutches, walker).
- Treat arthritis to improve mobility.
- Look out for hidden steps, wax, spills, grease, or water.
- Don't carry heavy or awkward objects.
- Don't carry objects in such a way that vision is obscured.
- Wear low, broad heels and nonskid footwear.
- Dress warmly.

Household Safety Tips

- Have all areas at home lighted with fluorescent or glazed bulbs.
- Do not use bare light bulbs (glare).
- Have lighting in stairwells and bathroom.
- Use nightlights, especially between bedroom and bathroom.
- Have light switches outside of each room; use illuminated light switches.
- Have handrails on both sides of wall of stairs indoors.
- Have handrails on front and back steps to the house and near the tub, shower, and toilet.
- Avoid slippery (waxed) linoleum, loose carpets, scattered toys, and pets. Use a waxless cleanser.
- Correct irregularities in floors.
- Clean spills quickly to avoid slipping.
- Remove unneeded low-lying objects from all rooms; don't leave objects on stairs.
- Don't climb over obstacles.
- Keep a sturdy step stool for reaching high places.
- Ensure that stairs and handrails are sound.
- Avoid throw rugs and frayed carpet or shag rugs.
- Beware of low beds and toilets.
- Be sure water drainage is adequate to prevent slippery floors after bathing.
- Don't leave objects on the floor.
- Seat height should be adequate for rising and sitting.
- Use a high chair for doing the dishes.
- Do not use slippers or shoes with slippery soles.
- Chairs must be stable and have arms.
- Avoid walking on ice and high curbs.
- Have walkways shoveled in the winter so they are free of ice or snow; have salt and sand available for slippery surfaces.
- Don't walk on uneven pavement.
- Have safety treads in bathtub.
- Have grasp bars on walls where you need them.
- Train pets not to jump on you.
- Place shelves within reach or use a reaching device.
- Position the telephones so that you do not have to hurry to answer them.
- Have a bedside table for such things as glasses rather than placing objects on the floor beside the bed.

The following booklets can be obtained free of charge from the American Association of Retired Persons, Fulfillment, 1909 K Street NW, Washington, DC 20049: *Do-Able, Renewable Home* and *Falling! The Unexpected Trip.*

Reexamine your home for potential areas where you may injure your spine. Install an automatic garage door opener. Keep window casings clean and lubricated. Use a pry bar to loosen stuck windows. Use a "reach" to pick up light objects. A pizza shovel may be useful to move food around the kitchen.

Using a cane to provide greater stability will prevent many falls in elderly individuals. Unfortunately, in recent years most people in the United States have come to view canes as signs of invalidism and old age. Only in the past few years has the walking stick re-emerged as a fashionable accessory. A large number of cane styles are available, including a variety of gadget canes for a variety of purposes. Women's canes are 34 inches long and men's 36. The cane may need to be shortened to be comfortable. Think of the cane as a sign of distinction and elegance. Select several that are attractive. You will find many types of wood and a variety of handle materials. Choose walking sticks that are attractive to you and that are conversation pieces. Carry your cane as a symbol of style and determination, not as a symbol of disability.

HOW TO AVOID INJURY TO THE SPINE

The architecture of the spine is arranged to minimize the effect of bearing weight. Maintaining good posture protects your spine from fracture and also protects the disks, the tissue between your vertebrae that behaves like shock absorbers. The upper back should be flat, whereas the lower back should arch backward. The shoulders should be back and pinched together toward each other. The head should be held high with the chin tucked in.

Maintain Good Posture

Once you have had a compression fracture of the spine, it becomes difficult to maintain good posture. As a result of fractures, the natural curve of the spine changes so that the upper back is curved, the head slumps forward, and the shoulders become rounded. This posture is undesirable not only because it is unattractive but also because it does not properly distribute forces placed on your spine (see Figure 4.2).

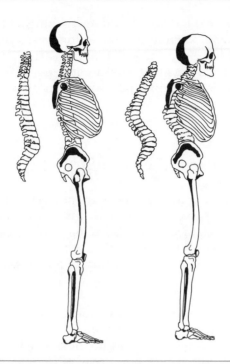

Figure 4.2 The change in posture that occurs as a result of osteoporotic fractures of the spine.

The front of your vertebrae is less protected from stress than is the back and is more subject to compression. The "natural" posture that follows a compression fracture results in more stress to the front of your vertebrae. Flexion of the spine does the same thing. The principles of avoiding vertebral fracture in the osteoporotic woman, then, include maintaining good posture and avoiding *spinal flexion*.

You must consciously maintain proper posture when lifting, pushing, or pulling. Always avoid flexing the spine in these activities; keep your back straight. When lifting an object, first test its weight so that you are sure you can handle it. Bend at the knees, maintaining the natural curve of your lower body. Keep the object close to your body. If you keep the object far out in front, you will be forced to flex your spine. Keep your feet flat and apart (about the width of your shoulders) to distribute your weight evenly between all the joints of the legs. Never bend at the waist to pick things up from the floor. Take a deep breath as you start to bend.

When pushing and pulling, change your normal motion so that you do not stoop. Bend at the knees, keeping your back straight, and move your feet forward and backward or from side to side as you might do while dancing. This is the rocking foot-to-foot motion you should use while vacuuming, sweeping, or raking the yard. This motion avoids bending at the waist and twisting. If you must work on the floor or ground, as when gardening, avoid flexing the spine by working in a half-kneeling position or on all fours using a box to support your body.

Devices to Prevent Spinal Injury

It may be helpful to know that there are devices designed to reduce or eliminate spinal flexion. The following is a list of devices available through either the Sears Specilog, *Home Health Care*, or through the *Mature Wisdom* catalog. Physicians, physical therapists, occupational therapists, and nurses may want to recommend these devices:

- toilet-seat riser—This 4-inch comfortable riser reduces strain from bending to a low toilet seat.
- reacher—This 32-inch aluminum device will pick up pieces of paper and so on. There is no reason to bend over.
- sock valet—Slide this contoured plastic sheet into your hosiery. The long fabric straps let you pull sock or stocking over your foot while you sit straight back.
- tub safety seat—This adjustable seat makes getting in and out of the bathtub easier.
- chair pad—Many chairs are either too low or hard, but this 3-inch cushion makes any seat easier to rest on.
- cane holder—This pocket-size holder clips to all canes so they will grip to an edge and not fall on the floor.
- cane hand loop—Nylon webbing is attached to a cane with Velcro fasteners.
- easy-lift pet tray—This attractive plastic tray holds two bowls attached to a 22-inch-long handle. You don't need to bend over to feed your cat or dog.
- shoehorn—This 23-inch shoehorn is designed to preclude bending.

As health professionals become more aware of the devices that can expand their patients' limited functioning, they will be better prepared to help them adjust to the lifestyle changes that will be necessary.

A LIFELONG STRATEGY FOR PREVENTING OSTEOPOROTIC FRACTURES

Preventing osteoporotic fractures is a lifelong battle against several changeable risk factors. It is important to realize that the incidence of hip fracture begins to rise in the decade before menopause and that a substantial amount of bone loss occurs from the spine and the femur prior to menopause. Prevention of osteoporosis must begin in childhood.

Behavior that promotes skeletal health includes all the dos and don'ts a mother teaches: "Do drink milk, eat a well-balanced diet, exercise regularly and sensibly, and play in the sunshine. Don't smoke cigarettes or drink alcohol or coffee." Heredity, nutrition, and exercise are probably the most important factors in achieving maximal peak bone mass in adulthood. At the time of menopause, an assessment of a woman's risk for developing osteoporosis will help determine whether she should undergo estrogen-replacement therapy. In later life, the tendency to fall becomes critical and must be minimized, and an adequate intake of vitamin D is important. A lifelong approach to preventing osteoporotic fractures is outlined in the shaded boxed area on the next page.

In the following chapters, specific information will be provided on nutrition, exercise, and estrogen-replacement therapy. Remember, however, that recommendations for preventing osteoporosis may not always apply to its treatment (and may even be dangerous for those who have established osteoporosis).

SUMMARY

Minimizing the risk of injury to the spine is as important as maximizing bone strength in preventing osteoporotic fractures. About half the falls in the elderly occur from tripping. They are more susceptible to tripping because of difficulty in correcting balance, changes in gait, visual loss, an impaired sense of balance, and decreased alertness. The remaining half of falls in the elderly result from suddenly falling to the ground. Falls are common because of drop attacks, loss of balance, and syncope.

Successful fall prevention requires attention to both the health factors that increase an individual's tendency to fall and the individual's immediate environment. Individuals with osteoporosis can minimize spinal injury by practicing correct posture in lifting, pushing, and pulling. They must also avoid flexion of the spine (bending forward at the waist). A number of helpful devices may also help prevent spinal injury. Finally, a lifelong strategy of prevention includes maximizing bone strength and minimizing the chances of injury.

A Lifelong Approach to Prevention of Osteoporotic Fractures

Childhood and Premenopausal Years

- Encourage weight-bearing exercise as well as exercise to improve coordination and flexibility.
- Establish other lifelong wellness habits:
    Avoid alcohol and tobacco.
    Avoid bone-robbing drugs.
    Include dairy products with each meal.
    Practice good posture.

Menopause

- Undergo hormonal replacement therapy if historical risk factors or low bone density is present.
- Review nutritional habits to be sure intake of calcium is adequate.
- Promote wellness (smoking and alcohol cessation).
- Continue weight-bearing exercise that also improves coordination and flexibility.

Elderly

- Exercise to promote agility.
- Encourage walking.
- Concentrate on health factors that affect the tendency to fall (hearing, vision, medications).
- Avoid spinal injury.
- Practice home safety.
- Assess nutritional status.
- Consider vitamin D supplementation.

5 CHAPTER

Osteoporosis and the Calcium Craze

We need an ample amount of dietary calcium to build strong bones in childhood and early adulthood and to prevent the bone loss that occurs with aging. The specific amount of calcium, as well as other nutrients, that we need has been determined by the Committee on Dietary Allowances of the Food and Nutrition Board. These amounts are called recommended dietary allowances (RDAs), which are the intake levels of essential nutrients that the Committee of Dietary Allowances of the Food and Nutrition Board considers to be adequate to meet the nutritional needs of almost all healthy persons. The RDA for calcium is 800 milligrams per day for adults and 1,200 milligrams per day for adolescents and pregnant and lactating women. Table 5.1 lists the RDA for calcium for the different stages of life.

Table 5.1   RDA for Calcium Throughout Life

Life stages	Age (yrs)	RDA (mg)
Infants	0-0.5	360
	0.5-1.0	540
Children	1-10	800
Adolescents	10-18	1,200
Adults	19 and older	800
Pregnant or lactating women	19 and older	1,200
	Under 19	1,600
Postmenopausal women	. . .	800

Although the RDAs are accepted as general guidelines, problems arise when attempting to apply them to a diverse population. For example, many scientists have pointed out that using the same RDA for both men and women may be inadvisable. They have questioned the validity of the RDA, pointing to studies that implicate dietary calcium deficiency in bone loss in women. In addition, the Food and Nutrition Board continues to recommend the same levels of calcium that it first set in 1941 despite advances in our knowledge of the relationship between calcium and bone loss.

Data from the most recent National Health and Nutrition Examination Survey (HANES II) conducted by the U.S. Department of Health and Human Services from 1976 to 1980 revealed that less than 33% of women between the ages of 18 and 74 met the RDA of 800 milligrams for calcium. Less than 25% of women over 35 met the RDA. On average, menopausal women took in only 514 milligrams a day. It's clear from this survey that calcium intake was low in the late 1970s. The next dietary survey will probably show an increase in calcium intake as a result of the recent obsession with calcium that has arisen in the United States. This chapter talks about the calcium craze and the use of calcium supplements in preventing osteoporosis.

WHAT IS THE CALCIUM CRAZE?

The calcium craze was the direct result of two things: (a) scientists' trying to inform the public about the role of low calcium intake in the development of osteoporosis, and (b) massive advertising of calcium supplements and products by the food and pharmaceutical industries. In 1982, members of the American Society of Bone and Mineral Research held a press conference following their annual meeting. Reporters were captivated by the thought that a disabling public health problem could be prevented simply by increasing the dietary intake of calcium. Then, in April 1984 the recommendations of the National Institutes of Health consensus panel concerning calcium intake were widely publicized. The panel recommended that postmenopausal women who were not taking estrogen should increase their calcium intake to 1,500 milligrams per day. Other publicized studies suggested that calcium may protect against high blood pressure and colon cancer.

Following this news, pharmaceutical firms rushed to manufacture and market calcium supplements—calcium had become the "miracle mineral" almost overnight. Proof that these marketing strategies were effective is revealed in an increase in sales of calcium supplements to $165 million per year by 1986; in 1987, sales were predicted to reach $200 million. The sales were fueled by advertisements that featured elderly women with stooped posture. One pharmaceutical firm spends $5 million on advertising its calcium supplement. The most dramatic example of the calcium craze was the result of a decision by the manufacturer of Tums antacids to redirect its $7-million campaign from Tums as an antacid to Tums as a calcium supplement—sales increased by 40% in 1985.

Food manufacturers soon joined the pharmaceutical firms in trying to capture the growing market by developing calcium-enriched products. By the beginning of 1987, consumers could find 25 calcium-enriched foods on grocery store shelves and in the frozen food section. It seems like every trip to the store reveals a new product fortified with calcium.

All this advertising has indeed increased public awareness of osteoporosis. Unfortunately, many women have been led to believe that by swallowing a calcium supplement they are completely protected from developing osteoporosis. Another problem with the calcium craze is that some people take too much calcium, believing that more is better.

THE EVIDENCE FOR INCREASING DIETARY INTAKE OF CALCIUM

The suggestion to increase calcium intake comes from several lines of evidence. Osteoporosis can be produced in laboratory animals by depriving them of calcium. One study from Yugoslavia (Matkovic et al., 1979) showed that women living in a region that had a high intake of dairy products had half the number of hip fractures as had women living in a district that consumed less dairy products. There is also evidence from several studies of an interaction of calcium intake with exercise and estrogen therapy. The studies suggest that exercise increases bone mass only when calcium intake is adequate and that the usual dose of estrogen that prevents bone loss may be reduced if calcium intake is high.

The recommendations for increasing calcium intake in postmenopausal women are primarily based on research performed at Creighton University in Omaha, Nebraska, on women eating their customary diets. Studies showed that the average calcium intake associated with zero calcium balance was about 500 milligrams higher in postmenopausal women than in premenopausal women

(Heaney, Recker, & Saville, 1977). (Remember that zero balance indicates that calcium is neither gained nor lost from the body.)

Ordinarily, this type of evidence is considered suggestive rather than definitive for a variety of reasons. To prove definitively that increasing dietary calcium is beneficial requires a clinical trial in which (a) bone mass is measured, (b) postmenopausal women are assigned at random either to a *placebo* (a pill that has no active ingredients) or to a calcium supplement group, and (c) the two groups are then compared to see whether the increased calcium did indeed prevent bone loss. Several studies of this type had actually been completed at the time of the National Institutes of Health consensus conference. The first, done by the Creighton researchers (Recker, Saville, & Heaney, 1977), suggested a benefit; another study was equivocal (Horsman, Gallagher, Simpson, & Nordin, 1977); and a third study (performed in Denmark) showed no benefit from calcium supplementation (Nilas, Christiansen, & Rodbro, 1984). Of special importance in the Danish study is that one group of women received estrogen and did not lose bone mass. Moreover, two additional clinical trials were presented at the June 1986 meeting of the American Society for Bone and Mineral Research. Both concluded that calcium supplementation was not as effective as estrogens were in preventing postmenopausal bone loss. One of these studies (Riis, Thomsen, & Christiansen, 1987) suggested that calcium supplementation may have a protective effect on loss of cortical bone, but no protective effect on loss of trabecular bone from the spine.

Are there other benefits to increasing calcium intake? There is evidence that a higher calcium intake may be protective against cancer of the colon, reduce blood pressure, and limit the damage done by periodontal disease. Calcium supplements reduced the growth rate of intestinal cells in people with a family history of cancer of the colon. Individuals with a low calcium intake have higher blood pressure than those with a high calcium intake, and studies concerning the use of supplements to lower blood pressure are being conducted in several research centers. Although a calcium-deficient diet does not cause periodontal disease, it may worsen its effects. Following dental extraction necessitated by periodontal disease, bone loss from the jaw may result in dentures fitting improperly. This bone loss may be reduced if calcium intake is increased. These potential benefits of increasing calcium intake require a great deal of additional research before sweeping recommendations can be made to the general population.

Let us try to put the calcium craze in perspective. Calcium is not a miracle mineral. However, ample calcium intake is important in developing maximal peak bone mass. A calcium intake of 1,500 milligrams per day is not as effective as estrogen is in preventing postmenopausal bone loss. One study (Heaney & Recker, 1986) suggested that as many as 25% of estrogen-deprived post-menopausal women will remain in negative calcium balance no matter how much calcium they ingest. Increasing dietary calcium intake alone will not protect all women from osteoporosis.

Remember that dietary calcium deficiency is only one of many risk factors for osteoporosis. Several other risk factors are proba-bly more powerful in their effect than is dietary calcium deficiency. If you have many risk factors for osteoporosis, it is not likely that taking calcium supplements alone will prevent osteoporosis. If a postmenopausal woman is taking estrogens, there is no reason to take more than 1,000 to 1,200 milligrams of calcium per day unless her physician prescribes a lower-than-usual dose of estro-gen. Should you take 1,500 milligrams of calcium per day? Until there is more information, this amount is recommended for post-menopausal women who are at high risk of osteoporosis but who decide not to take estrogen.

You do not need to become obsessed with your calcium intake. On the other hand, you should not have a calcium-deficient diet. With planning you can ensure a dietary calcium intake of 1,200 or even 1,500 milligrams per day. If you are on a low-calcium diet, raise your dietary intake by including a dairy product with each meal. Food is preferable to calcium supplements. However, if you decide to take supplements, simplify this process also. The less elaborate the meal plans and calcium supplementation, the more likely you will succeed in accomplishing your goal for calcium intake. Information to help you plan a calcium-rich diet is provided in chapter 6. In the remainder of this chapter, the use of calcium supplementation will be discussed.

WHAT ABOUT CALCIUM SUPPLEMENTS?

The sale of calcium supplements is not subject to the same degree of regulation as are medications by the Food and Drug Adminis-tration. Many different supplements have been placed on the market without the scrutiny to which drugs are normally subjected. Also, there is little information concerning the *bioavailability* and long-term safety of these products. Bioavailability refers to the fact that different forms of the same chemical may produce varied effects

in the body depending on how they are processed. Thus, it is possible that different amounts of calcium will be absorbed depending on whether a capsule or a tablet is used or whether there is a
high or low amount of calcium in the tablet (or per dose). Only
recently has calcium supplementation been studied in detail. The
safety of calcium supplementation will undoubtedly be determined
in the next several years.

WHICH CALCIUM SUPPLEMENT IS BEST?

There is a confusing array of calcium supplements available over
the counter. A sample of the variety currently on the market is
shown in Table 5.2, which groups calcium supplements according
to the source of the calcium in the product.

Calcium is not present in a free form but is combined with other
substances to form a compound. Calcium carbonate, the preferred
calcium source, is obtained from oyster shell. Egg shell also serves
as a source. Most people raised an incredulous eyebrow when it was
suggested that one of the cheapest forms of calcium is Tums (which
is not prescribed for the "tummy"). Tums are calcium carbonate
and may be recommended as a calcium supplement. Tribasic and
Dibasic calcium phosphate are generally not recommended because
there is plenty of phosphorus in the American diet. However, no
studies have been done to examine whether calcium phosphate is
better or worse than calcium carbonate. Bonemeal or dolomite are
not recommended as calcium sources because they may contain
other substances (such as lead) that may be harmful. The amount
of lead in these products might not be toxic, but, because there is
no strict FDA rule, you cannot be certain that the level of lead is
safe. Also, be aware of the term "low lead" on the supplement label.
Here again, there are no government regulations on lead levels. Calcium lactate often causes an upset stomach. Calcium gluconate is
a calcium supplement that has few undesirable side effects. Calcium glubionate is available as a liquid for those who do not want
to swallow tablets.

An interesting form of calcium that has recently been studied is
calcium citrate. Unlike calcium carbonate, this form is absorbed
even when reduced gastric (stomach) acid secretion is a problem.
Thus, calcium citrate is more predictable than is calcium carbonate
in terms of the amount of calcium absorbed, particularly in the
elderly, who may have reduced stomach acid levels. Moreover, the

Table 5.2 Over-the-Counter Calcium Supplements

Product name (manufacturer)	Elemental calcium/tablet (approx. mg)	Calcium compound/tablet (approx. mg)	Cost index[a] (cost/100 mg elemental calcium)
Calcium carbonate			
Caltrate 600 (Lederle)	600	1,500	34
Gencalc 600 (Goldline)	600	1,500	10
Suplical (Warner-Lambert)	600	1,500	40
Super Calcium 1200 (Schiff)	600	1,512	..
Calcium carbonate (various brands)	600	1,500	..
Biocal (Miles)	500	1,250	29
Oscal 500 (Marion)	500	1,250	42
Oyst-Cal 500 (Goldline)	500	1,250	14
Oyster-Cal 500 (Natures Bounty)	500	1,250	14
Cal-Sup (Riker)	300	750	37
Calciday 667 (Nature's Bounty)	267	667	24
Calcium carbonate (various brands)	260	650	34+
Biocal (Miles), chewable	250	625	57
Os-Cal 250 (Marion)	250	625	..

(Cont.)

Table 5.2 (Continued)

Product name (manufacturer)	Elemental calcium/tablet (approx. mg)	Calcium compound/tablet (approx. mg)	Cost index[a] (cost/100 mg elemental calcium)
Calcium carbonate			
Florical (Mericon) (contains 8.3 mg sodium fluoride)	146	364	104
Ca-Plus Protein (Miller)	112	280	29
Elecal (Western Research) (contains 15 mg magnesium)	100	250	17
Antacids containing calcium carbonate			
Alka Mints, chewable (Miles)	340	850	103
Tums, extra strength, chewable (Norcliff-Thayer)	300	750	128
Calcium carbonate (various brands) tablets	260	650	56+
Tums, regular chewable (Norcliff-Thayer)	200	500	42
Chooz (Plough), chewable	200	500	131
Dicarbosil, chewable (Norcliff-Thayer)	200	500	72
Equilet, chewable (Mission Pharmaceutical)	200	500	46
Mallamint, chewable (Mallant)	168	420	48
Amitone, chewable (Norcliff-Thayer)	140	350	51

Calcium carbonate with vitamin D

Caltrate 600 with vitamin D 125 IU vitamin D/tablet (Lederle)	600	1,500	202
Caltrate 600 with vitamin D plus iron 125 IU with iron/tablet (Lederle)	600	1,500	232
Os-Cal 250 tablet (Marion)	250	625	37
Oyst-Cal-D tabs (Goldline)	250	625	33
Oystercal-D 250 tablets (Nature's Bounty)	250	625	42

Tribasic Calcium Phosphate

Posture (Ayerst)	235	600	28
Posture (Ayerst)	117	300	28

Tribasic calcium phosphate with vitamin D

Posture-D tablets (Ayerst)	600	1,540	170
Posture-D tablets (Ayerst)	300	770	108

Dibasic calcium phosphate

Dibasic calcium phosphate (Lilly)	112	486	38

Dibasic calcium phosphate with vitamin D

Dibasic calcium phosphate with vitamin D pulvules (Lilly)	116	400	85

Table 5.2 (Continued)

Product name (manufacturer)	Elemental calcium/tablet (approx. mg)	Calcium compound/tablet (approx. mg)	Cost index[a] (cost/100 mg elemental calcium)
Calcium lactate			
Calcium lactate (various brands: Lilly, GNC, CUS, Thompson, Texall, Food Center, Nature's Bounty)	85	650	28
Calcium lactate (various brands)	42	325	47
Calcium citrate			
Citracal (Mission Pharmaceutical)	200	950	...
Calcium gluconate			
Calcium gluconate (various brands)	90	1,000	50+
	58	650	41+
	45	500	84+
Calcium gluconate with vitamin D			
Calcium gluconate with vitamin D tablets (Lilly)	93	1,034	255
Calcium gluconate with vitamin D pulvules (Lilly)	30	334	163

	Calcium glubionate 115/5 ml syrup	1,800/5 ml syrup	166
Neo-Calglucon (Sandoz)			

[a]The cost index is a ratio of the average wholesale prices for equivalent quantities of a drug. The cost indexes for dosage forms of different strengths are adjusted to compare equivalent amounts of products accurately. As an example of the cost index, if Product A has a cost index of 15, and Product B has a cost index of 45, Product A is 3 times as expensive as Product B (based on average wholesale cost). The cost index is only an indication of relative wholesale costs and is not a rating or recommendation. It is based only on average wholesale price and is presented for information purposes only without consideration of potential differences in the quality of similar products.

Sources—E.K. Kastovp (Ed.) (1986). *Drug Facts and Comparison* (1986 ed.). St. Louis: Facts and Comparisons (division of J.B. Lippincott).

citrate form may be protective against the formation of calcium-rich kidney stones. Calcium citrate became available in 1986. Anyone with any form of kidney disease should not take calcium without first consulting a physician.

WHAT IS ELEMENTAL CALCIUM?

The substances to which calcium is bound in a compound usually constitute the majority of the weight of the calcium source. When buying a calcium supplement, look at the amount of calcium in the compound, not the weight of the entire compound. This is referred to as *elemental* (or actual) *calcium*. Table 5.3 identifies the percentage of elemental calcium in various calcium sources. Elemental calcium refers to the actual amount of available calcium in a supplement and is measured in milligrams.

Remember that there are 1,000 milligrams in 1 gram. When calcium supplements list the number of milligrams per tablet, it is important to identify whether the manufacturer is referring to the milligrams of the entire calcium compound or only of the elemental calcium. If the amount of the calcium compound is being referred to, then Table 5.3 should be consulted to determine the percentage of elemental calcium in the compound.

Table 5.3   Elemental Calcium Contents of Various Sources

Calcium source	Percentage of elemental calcium
Calcium carbonate	40
Calcium sulfate	36
Tribasic calcium phosphate	39
Bonemeal	32
Dibasic calcium phosphate	29
Dolomite	22
Calcium lactate	13
Calcium ascorbate	10
Calcium gluconate	9
Calcium glubionate	6.5
Calcium citrate	24

Assume that a calcium supplement manufacturer states that each tablet supplies 600 milligrams of calcium carbonate. After referring to Table 5.3, you calculate that each 600-milligram tablet provides only 240 milligrams of elemental calcium as calcium carbonate is 40% calcium and 60% carbonate.

$$600 \text{ mg calcium carbonate} \times .40 \text{ mg calcium}$$
$$\approx 240 \text{ mg elemental calcium}$$

Therefore, if you calculate that you need to supplement your diet with 500 milligrams of elemental calcium and you purchase 600-milligram calcium carbonate tablets, you will need to take two 600-milligram calcium carbonate tablets to consume approximately 500 milligrams of elemental calcium.

$$240 \text{ mg elemental calcium per } 600 \text{ mg calcium carbonate}$$
$$\text{tablet} \times 2 \approx 480 \text{ mg elemental calcium}$$

As you can see in Table 5.3, some supplements have a small percentage of elemental calcium, making them impractical. For example, if you need 500 milligrams of calcium, you would need 11 or more 500-milligram tablets of calcium gluconate (9% calcium) compared to only two 600-milligram tablets of calcium carbonate (40% calcium). To avoid confusion, more companies now list the amount of elemental calcium. The recently released calcium citrate products warrant special attention. More of the compound is absorbed than any of the other supplements. As a result, if you have a goal of obtaining 1,000 or 1,500 milligrams of calcium, only 600 to 800 milligrams of calcium citrate is needed.

Comparison shop for the least expensive calcium supplements. This involves reading the labels. You must compare the cost per milligram of elemental calcium. A recent survey revealed the following cost differential (wholesale prices) for 500 milligrams of calcium: 5 cents for generic oyster shell, 6 cents for Tums, 10 cents for Oscal-500, and $1.40 for calcium gluconate (which contains only 49 milligrams of calcium per pill). Table 5.2 also gives cost index information for certain calcium supplements.

CALCIUM SUPPLEMENTS AND BIOAVAILABILITY

Remember, however, that the Food and Drug Administration (FDA) has not required manufacturers of calcium supplements to demonstrate the bioavailability of their products. Enteric-coated calcium carbonate, for example, does not dissolve in the stomach and is not absorbed adequately. A special conference on osteoporosis was held by the Food and Drug Administration in October 1987. At that conference Dr. Ralph F. Shangraw of the University of Maryland reported on his studies of calcium supplements. He tested more than 80 of the calcium carbonate supplements on the market and found that the effectiveness of more than half of them was questionable. He used the standard established by the United States Pharmacopeia for disintegration and dissolution. Disintegration indicates that the tablet breaks up into small particles; dissolution means it dissolves into molecules. Tablets must disintegrate within 30 minutes, and 75% of the tablet should be dissolved in that time. Disintegration is easy to test—if your tablets do not disintegrate they are not useful.

Many companies are reformulating their products so that they will disintegrate. While waiting for these companies to respond, you can do a home test on your calcium carbonate tablets. Place the tablet in a 6 oz glass of white vinegar at room temperature. Stir every few minutes. In 30 minutes the tablet should have disintegrated. If it has not you should change supplements.

SHOULD CALCIUM SUPPLEMENTS CONTAIN OTHER MINERALS AND VITAMINS?

Individuals who consume primarily commercially processed foods could be magnesium deficient since magnesium is removed in processing. Alcoholism, uncontrolled diabetes, and certain diuretics also can cause magnesium deficiency. However, magnesium is found in many foods, including green vegetables, seafood, milk, nuts, and whole grains, and there is no evidence for a beneficial effect of magnesium in amounts exceeding the RDA of 300 to 400 milligrams per day. Therefore, few people would need more magnesium than can be obtained from a normal diet, and calcium supplements do not need to contain magnesium. Dolomite has been popular because of the mistaken belief that magnesium should be present in calcium supplements, but dolomite also contains cadmium, uranium, arsenic, and lead.

There is no reason to add iron or vitamin C to calcium supplements as they do not enhance calcium absorption. Take calcium supplements separately from iron pills because calcium carbonate may reduce iron absorption. If you want to take calcium, there is no rationale for using a so called natural source or a preparation that includes minerals of no known value in enhancing calcium absorption. The calcium in Tums is as "natural" as the calcium in dolomite. Some advertising refers to *chelated calcium*. There is no proven advantage of using chelated calcium. The same is true of *conatural supplements*, which are a combination of synthetic and natural forms.

WHEN SHOULD CALCIUM SUPPLEMENTS BE TAKEN?

The time of day that you take calcium may have some importance. Postmenopausal women seem to lose calcium during sleep, when they are not eating. Therefore, some researchers have recommended that calcium be taken before bedtime. Recent studies have shown, however, that calcium carbonate is not absorbed on an empty stomach in patients who have low levels of stomach acid. This is the case in many older women, who should take the supplement immediately after eating so that it will be absorbed. Moreover, some women develop gastrointestinal symptoms from calcium supplements, such as nausea, bloating, gaseousness, and sometimes changes in bowel habits (diarrhea or constipation). These symptoms frequently subside when calcium is taken with meals. Calcium supplements should be taken in divided doses with meals. If low levels of stomach acid are not a problem or if calcium citrate is used, some of the calcium may be taken at bedtime.

CAN CALCIUM SUPPLEMENTATION BE HARMFUL?

The concept of "too much of a good thing" must be applied to calcium supplementation. Many individuals take an excess of calcium because they believe that more is better. Others mistakenly believe that they require 1,500 milligrams of calcium supplementation in addition to their dietary intake. This is a dangerous practice that can result in a high level of calcium in the blood or urine.

A number of years ago, when calcium compounds were used widely as antacids, a condition called the *milk-alkali syndrome* was observed. Patients who took large amounts of milk and calcium carbonate developed high blood calcium levels, deposits of calcium in tissues outside of bone, and even renal failure. There are enough nonabsorbable antacids (and other drugs) available that milk-alkali syndrome rarely occurs now. However, with uninformed, injudicious use of calcium and vitamin D, similar problems in the near future may arise.

On the other hand, most physicians consider a calcium intake up to 2,500 to 3,000 milligrams per day as safe. Proponents of a high calcium intake remind us that calcium intake in Western civilizations is comparatively low. For example, prehistoric man consumed 1,600 to 2,700 milligrams per day. Contemporary African Masai warriors actually ingest 6,000 milligrams of calcium daily. And in America 10 percent of young males consume over 2,200 milligrams of calcium a day.

The major concern about higher calcium intakes is the potential for kidney stones. Yet increasing calcium intake by 1,000 milligrams will increase urinary calcium levels by only 60 milligrams per day. Furthermore, dietary calcium does not cause kidney stones. Increased risk for kidney stones occurs only in those individuals who have a predisposition toward developing them.

Be careful to take an adequate but not an excessive amount of calcium supplements. If you or any member of your family has kidney stones, do not take calcium supplements without a physician's supervision. There may be an advantage of using calcium citrate if you have had stones because citrate is protective against stone formation. On the other hand, if you have not had kidney stones and do not have a family history of kidney stones, do not be overly concerned with occasionally consuming a slight excess of calcium. Be certain to drink plenty of liquids if you take calcium supplements. Maintaining a daily urine volume of 2 liters helps protect against the development of kidney stones. Taking the supplement with a glass of water, milk, or juice will also improve its absorption.

Your physician may ask you to take a test that measures the calcium content in a 24-hour collection of urine. If you are absorbing more calcium than your bones use in bone formation, the excess is excreted in the urine. Calcium deposits in areas such as the *bursae* (bursitis) do *not* result from excess calcium intake; rather, calcium deposits in inflamed tissues are a response to tissue injury.

SUMMARY

Our bodies need an adequate amount of calcium to develop strong, healthy skeletons (peak bone mass). Adequate calcium is also needed so that exercise and estrogens can promote skeletal health. The growing consensus is that the RDA for calcium is too low and should be increased to 1,000 to 1,200 milligrams; postmenopausal women who are not taking estrogen should increase their intake to 1,500 milligrams.

However, calcium is not a miracle mineral. It is not as effective as estrogen in preventing postmenopausal bone loss. More important, you need to see calcium as interacting with other factors that influence skeletal mass rather than as a cure-all for preventing osteoporosis.

The best strategy is to obtain calcium from food sources as often as you can. If you find this difficult because of food preferences or intolerance, calcium supplements may be more convenient. Choose an effective and inexpensive supplement. Also, remember that the recommendations for calcium intake include calcium obtained through both diet and supplements—don't take an excessive amount of calcium. The next chapter provides detailed information on eating for skeletal health.

6 CHAPTER

Preventing Osteoporosis Through Proper Nutrition

Simply telling you to increase your intake of dietary calcium would be inadequate without providing further background information about nutrition. Good nutrition depends on eating a well-balanced diet rather than focusing on consuming one particular nutrient. For instance, if you increase your calcium intake by adding foods with a high fat and cholesterol content, you could gain too much weight and/or increase your blood cholesterol level. In this case, a well-intentioned change in your diet could lead to undesirable effects on your health. You should strive for balance in the foods you eat. This chapter reviews basic nutritional principles and tells you how to eat for skeletal health.

NEW AMERICAN DIETARY GOALS

Our society is plagued by obesity and a number of other lifestyle diseases—heart disease, high blood pressure, diabetes, cirrhosis of the liver, and even osteoporosis—that are directly related to eating and health habits.

Since the turn of the century, our eating habits have changed dramatically. Today, we consume less milk and fresh fruit and fewer grain products and fresh vegetables and much more fat, soft drinks, sugar, and alcohol than ever before. Our total caloric intake has dropped slightly, but, because we are significantly less active than our ancestors as a result of all our modern conveniences, we are heavier.

In response to this general decline in our eating habits, dietary goals have been established to improve the health of our nation. In 1977, George McGovern led the Senate Select Committee on

Nutrition and Human Needs in an extensive investigation of the dietary habits of Americans. The committee recommended we consume less fat, especially less artery-clogging saturated fat and cholesterol, less refined and processed sugars, fewer calories, and more complex carbohydrates and fiber. The U.S. Department of Agriculture and U.S. Department of Health and Human Services summarized these recommendations in its publication "Nutrition and Your Health: Dietary Guidelines for Americans." Let's take a closer look at these dietary guidelines.

DIETARY GUIDELINES

When planning to increase the calcium content of your diet you should keep the following guidelines in mind.

- **Eat a variety of foods.** The typical American diet generally relies on a few standard foods. You should strive to include a variety of vegetables, fruits, whole-grain breads and cereals, dairy products, meats, and other protein sources such as fish, egg, beans, and peas.
- **Maintain a desirable weight.** Although ideal body-weight values have been increased in recent years, obesity is still a major public health problem in the United States. It is clear that obesity can lead to high blood pressure, heart disease, and diabetes. The Center for Science in the Public Interest has devised a chart, shown in Table 6.1, that categorizes foods as to how they can be consumed following the USDA/USDHHS Dietary Guidelines. Foods in the "Anytime" category are less than 30% fat and generally are low in sugar and saturated fat. "In moderation" foods have moderate amounts of "good" polyunsaturated fatty acids (see below) or low to intermediate amounts of saturated fat. "Now and then" foods contain large amounts of saturated fat, and at least 50% of their calories are derived from fat.

  Osteoporosis is one health problem that is associated with thinness rather than obesity. One reason for this is that estrogens not only are manufactured in the ovaries but also are produced to some extent in fat tissue. Postmenopausal women who weigh more produce more estrogen than postmenopausal women who are less heavy, so even though ovarian estrogen in both groups is equally low, heavier women get an estrogen boost from their fat cells.

Severe thinness in young girls may produce estrogen deficiency, again because the low number of fat cells results in low estrogen contribution from this source. The serious eating disorder of anorexia nervosa is associated with the development of osteoporosis. The association of osteoporosis with elite distance runners who develop estrogen deficiency is also related to their low caloric intake and fat levels.

- **Avoid too much fat, saturated fat, and cholesterol.** Fat is a calorically dense nutrient with more than twice the number of calories of either carbohydrate or protein. The various types of fat in fat-containing foods affect the blood cholesterol level. Saturated fats, which are found in all foods of animal origin and in coconut and palm oils, raise blood cholesterol levels. Polyunsaturated fats, found in vegetable oils, tend to lower blood cholesterol levels. Olive oil is a monounsaturated fat and has become popular for its protective effect against heart disease.

Cholesterol is an important substance that is produced naturally by the body. There are several types of cholesterol in the blood. The important ones are *low-density lipoprotein* (LDL) and *high-density lipoprotein* (HDL). Low-density lipoprotein is known as the "bad" cholesterol. High levels of LDL in the bloodstream promote heart disease, whereas elevated levels of HDL are considered protective against heart disease. Olive oil appears to decrease the damaging LDL in the blood while still preserving the level of beneficial HDL. Although polyunsaturated fats lower the total cholesterol level, they seem to decrease both the LDL and the HDL levels. Therefore, a good diet will decrease the intake of saturated fats from animal products and include various vegetable oils and polyunsaturated fatty acids as well as olive oil. You should have your blood cholesterol level checked by your physician. Levels above 200 milligrams *may* require treatment. A healthy diet should limit the total fat content to 25% to 30% of the total calories and 250 to 300 milligrams of cholesterol per day. Avoid fatty cuts of meat by choosing poultry, fish, and lean cuts of meat. Substitute low-fat milk and cheese for whole milk and decrease consumption of eggs, butter, and other high-cholesterol foods such as liver. Strive to limit your intake of foods with a high total fat content and replace saturated fatty acids as much as possible with polyunsaturated fatty acids and olive oil. The New American Eating Guide (Table 6.1) will help you choose lower-fat foods.

Table 6.1   New American Eating Guide

Anytime	In Moderation	Now and Then
	Beans, Grains and Nuts (4 or more servings per day)	
Beans and peas, dried	Bread and rolls, white[8]	Cereals, presweetened[5, 8]
Bread and rolls, whole grain	Cereals, refined, unsweetend[8]	Croissants[4, 8]
Bulgar	Cornbread[8]	Doughnuts[3 or 4, 5, 8]
Cereals, whole grain, hot and cold	Flour tortillas[8]	Sticky buns[1 or 2, 5, 8]
Lentils	Granola cereals[1 or 2]	Stuffing, with butter[4, (6), 8]
Matzoh, whole wheat	Hominy grits[8]	
Oatmeal	Macaroni and cheese[1, (6), 8]	
Pasta, whole wheat	Matzoh[8]	
Rice, brown	Nuts[3]	
Sprouts	Pasta, except whole wheat[8]	
	Peanut butter[3]	
	Pizza[6, 8]	
	Refried beans[1 or 2]	
	Rice, white[8]	
	Seeds[3]	
	Soybeans[2]	

Tofu[2]

Waffles or pancakes, with syrup[5, (6), 8]

Fruits and Vegetables
(4 or more servings per day)

All fruits and vegetables except those at right	Avocado[3]	Coconut[4]
Applesauce, unsweetened	Carrots, glazed[5, (6)]	Pickles[6]
Fruit juices, unsweetened	Cole slaw[3]	
Potatoes, white or sweet	Cranberry sauce, canned[5]	
Vegetable juices, unsalted	Eggplant, fried in vegetable oil[2]	
	French fries, homemade in vegetable oil[2], commercial[2]	
	Fruit, canned in syrup[5]	
	Fruit, dried	
	Fruit juices, sweetened[5]	
	Gazpacho[2, (6)]	
	Guacamole[3]	
	Potatoes au gratin[1, (6)]	
	Vegetable juices, salted[6]	
	Vegetables, canned with salt[6]	

(Cont.)

Table 6.1 (Continued)

Anytime	In Moderation	Now and Then
	Milk Products	
	*(3-4 servings per day for children, 2 for adults)**	
Buttermilk, from skim milk	Cocoa from skim milk[5]	Cheesecake[4, 5]
Cheese, skim milk[6]	Cottage cheese, 4% milk fat[1]	Cheese fondue[4. (6)]
Cottage cheese, low fat	Ice milk[5]	Cheese soufflé[4. (6). 7]
Lassi (lowfat yogurt and fruit juice drink)	Milk, low-fat, 2% milk fat	Cheeses, hard; blue, brick, Camembert, cheddar, muenster,
Milk, low-fat, 1% milk fat	Mozzarella, part skim[1. (6)]	Swiss[4. (6)]
Milk, nonfat dry	Yogurt, low fat, frozen[5]	Cheeses, processed[4. 6]
Milk, skim	Yogurt, low fat, sweetened[5]	Eggnog[1. 5, 7]
Milk shake, skim milk and banana		Milk, whole[4]
Yogurt, low fat		Yogurt, whole milk[4]
	Poultry, Fish, Meat, and Eggs	
	(2 servings per day; vegetarians	
	should eat added servings from other groups)	
Chicken or turkey, boiled, baked, or roasted, without skin	Bacon[4. (6)]	Beef liver, fried[1. 7]
	Chicken, fried, homemade in vegetable oil[3]	Bologna[4. 6]
Cod		Chicken, fried, commercially

Egg, whites only
Flounder
Gefilte fish[(6)]
Haddock
Halibut
Perch
Pollock
Rockfish
Shellfish, except shrimp
Sole
Tuna, water-packed[(6)]

Chicken liver, baked or broiled (just one!)[7]
Chicken or turkey, broiled, baked, or roasted, with skin[2]
Fish, fried[1 or 2]
Flank steak, trimmed[1]
Herring[3, 6]
Lamb, leg or loin, trimmed[1]
Mackerel, canned[2, (6)]
Pork, shoulder or loin, lean, trimmed[1]
Round steak or ground round, trimmed[1]
Rump roast, trimmed[1]
Salmon, pink, canned[2, (6)]
Sardines[2, (6)]
Shrimp[7]
Sirloin steak, lean, trimmed[1]

prepared[4]
Corned beef[4, 6]
Egg, whole or yolk (about 3/week)[3, 7]
Ground beef[4]
Ham, trimmed[1, 6]
Hot dogs[4, 6]
Liverwurst[4, 6]
Omelet, cheese[4, 7]
Pig's feet[4]
Red meat, untrimmed[4]
Salami[4, 6]
Sausage[4, 6]
Spareribs[4]

(Cont.)

Table 6.1 (Continued)

Anytime	In Moderation	Now and Then
	Poultry, Fish, Meat, and Eggs	
	Tuna, oil-packed[2,6]	[6]May be high in salt or sodium
	Veal, trimmed[1]	[7]High in cholesterol
		[8]Refined grains

* Allowance based on basic four food group recommendations. Some individuals needing to increase their calcium intake may require more servings.

[1]Moderate fat, saturated   [4]High fat, saturated

[2]Moderate fat, unsaturated   [5]High in added sugar

[3]High fat, unsaturated   [6]High in salt or sodium

Reprinted from *New American Eating Guide* which is available from the Center for Science in the Public Interest, 1501 16th Street, N.W., Washington, D.C. 20036, for $3.95, copyright 1986.

- **Eat foods with adequate starch and fiber.** When you are lowering the total fat intake of your diet, it helps to eat more starch or complex carbohydrate to provide satiety. Complex carbohydrate or starch refers to whole-grain breads and cereals, pasta, legumes, beans, peas, and lentils. The complex carbohydrate food sources mentioned are for the most part also good sources of fiber. Insoluble fibers include bran, cellulose, lignin, and hemicellulose and are found primarily in raw vegetables, fruits, bran, and whole grains and cereals. Soluble fibers, including guar, pectin, and gums, are found primarily in beans, lentils, and legumes and oat bran. They are helpful in controlling the blood glucose level and in reducing blood cholesterol levels. It is recommended that one consume 25 to 35 grams of dietary fiber for every 1,000 calories consumed. There is no proven benefit in exceeding an intake of 50 grams of dietary fiber per day. In fact, excess fiber can decrease the amount of calcium absorbed from the diet. An increase in fiber of 25 to 35 grams may increase your calcium requirements by 150-200 mg per day.

- **Avoid too much sugar.** Sugar is an empty calorie nutrient that provides only calories and no vitamins or minerals. Because obesity is a problem for many, it is helpful to avoid an excessive intake of sugar and foods that contain sugar. It is also well known that sugar, especially sugary food eaten between meals, helps promote tooth decay. Recent attention has been given to studies showing that sugars increase calcium absorption. In actuality, this effect is not great; it is worthy of attention only for individuals with certain illnesses, such as diseases of the small intestine. Cut back on your sugar calories by eating fresh fruit instead of other sweet desserts or treats, and by eliminating soft drinks from your diet. Read ingredient labels on food packages to spot hidden sources of sugar and prepare food with less sugar.

- **Avoid too much sodium.** Americans also consume large amounts of sodium from convenience and processed foods. Other contributions of sodium come from sodium used in cooking and of course, the naturally occurring sodium in our foods. The average American consumes 10 to 20 grams of salt per day, equivalent to 2 to 4 teaspoons per day. The RDA for sodium for adults is 1,100 to 3,300 milligrams per day. Because table salt is 40% sodium and 60% chloride, this RDA is the equivalent of 3 to 8 grams, or approximately ½ to 1½ teaspoons of salt. Thus, Americans take in many times the recommended amount of sodium daily. An excess amount of sodium may be related to high blood pressure and may also cause urinary calcium loss.

The Dietary Guidelines for Americans encourage reducing salt intake to 5 grams per day. This is equivalent to 2,000 milligrams of sodium per day. Such a goal can be achieved by avoiding high-sodium food, by limiting the use of convenience and canned processed foods, by limiting salt in cooking and at the table, and by checking food labels for hidden sources of sodium. When checking nutrition labels on packages for sodium content, remember that this information is recorded in milligrams of sodium per serving. When cooking, leave out the salt and instead experiment with herbs and spices, onions, and fresh garlic or garlic powder for flavoring.

Two pamphlets that will help you lower your sodium intake are available free of charge from the U.S. Government Consumer Information Center: *A Word About Low Sodium Diets* (524R) and *Do Yourself a Flavor* (525R). Write to S. James, Consumer Information Center-D, P.O. Box 100, Pueblo, CO 81002.

- **If you drink alcohol, do so in moderation.** Alcohol contains many calories but provides almost no vitamins or minerals. Excessive alcohol intake may lead to obesity and liver disease, and alcoholism is associated with osteoporosis. However, one or two glasses of wine a day may provide some protection against heart attack. If you do drink alcohol, limit your intake to the equivalent of 2 ounces of hard liquor per day.

These guidelines are useful in maintaining health in the general population. They are particularly important for people who are at risk for osteoporosis.

ESTIMATING CALCIUM INTAKE

Each individual must determine how to meet daily calcium needs on the basis of personal food preferences, nutritional needs, and lifestyle. A calcium intake system that might work for one person may be unsuitable for another or may be unrealistic for some people on certain days of the week. Everyone should develop a simple plan for achieving a target daily calcium intake to ensure success. Developing such a plan begins with a knowledge of the foods that provide the most calcium (Table 6.2) and which of these foods you prefer. Information about the amount of calcium normally consumed during a typical day is also helpful.

Table 6.2   Calcium and Cholesterol Content of Foods

Food	Amount	Calcium (mg)	Cholesterol (mg)
Excellent Sources			
Dairy Products			
Yogurt, plain, low fat	8 ounces	415	14
Skim milk	8 ounces	302	4
1% milk	8 ounces	300	10
2% milk	8 ounces	297	18
Whole milk	8 ounces	290	33
Buttermilk	8 ounces	285	9
Chocolate milk	8 ounces	287	30
Nonfat, dry milk	1/3 cup	279	4
Swiss cheese	1 ounce	272	26
Cheddar cheese	1 ounce	204	30
Fish			
Sardines, canned with bones	3 ounces	372	120
Salmon, pink, canned, with bones	3 ounces	165	30
Very Good Sources			
Dairy Products			
Processed American cheese	1 ounce	174	27
Cheese foods	1 ounce	160	18
Cheese spread	1 ounce	159	16
Dessert			
Custard, baked	1/2 cup	150	138
Vegetable			
Turnip greens	1/2 cup cooked	184	0

(Cont.)

Table 6.2   (Continued)

Food	Amount	Calcium (mg)	Cholesterol (mg)
	Very Good Sources		
Vegetables			
Mustard greens	1/2 cup cooked	183	0
Collard greens	1/2 cup cooked	152	0
Dandelion greens	1/2 cup cooked	140	0
Kale	1/2 cup cooked	134	0
	Good Sources		
Dairy Products			
Vanilla ice cream	1/2 cup	88	30
Cottage cheese, 2% fat	1/2 cup	77	10
Cottage cheese, 1% fat	1/2 cup	69	5
Cottage cheese, creamed	1/2 cup	62	34
Desserts			
Pudding, made with whole milk	1/2 cup	132	16
Fish			
Clams, raw	3 ounces	47	43
Oysters, raw	1/2 cup (5 to 8 medium)	113	200
Shrimp, canned	3 ounces	98	128
Fruit			
Rhubarb	3/8 cup	78	0

Table 6.2   (Continued)

Food	Amount	Calcium (mg)	Cholesterol (mg)
	Good Sources		
Grain Product			
Waffle, homemade	7 ″ diameter	85	64
Nuts			
Almonds, dried, salted or unsalted	1/4 cup	76	0
Vegetables			
Beet greens	1/2 cup	99	0
Spinach	1/2 cup	98	0
Okra	1/2 cup	92	0
Broccoli	1/2 cup	68	0
	Poor Sources		
Cereals and Grains			
Pancake	4 ″ diameter	45	32
Biscuit	2 ″ diameter	42	15
Cereal, refined	1/2 cup cooked 3/4 cup dry	35	0
Bread, white	1 slice	21	0
Bread, wheat	1 slice	23	0
Macaroni, cooked	1/2 cup	8	0
Rice, cooked	1/2 cup	7	0
Saltines	2 ″ squares (5)	2	0

(Cont.)

Table 6.2   (Continued)

Food	Amount	Calcium (mg)	Cholesterol (mg)
	Poor Sources		
Desserts			
Candy, milk chocolate	1 ounce	52	2
Cake, white	2″ × 3″ × 3″	34	1
Pie, fruit	1/8 of 9″ pie	23	15
Honey	1 tablespoon	4	0
Fats			
French Dressing	1 tablespoon	2	10
Butter	1 teaspoon	1	11
Margarine	1 teaspoon	1	0
Mayonnaise	1 teaspoon	1	3
Fruit			
Fresh fruit	1/2 cup 1 medium	16	0
Canned fruit	1/2 cup	10	0
Fruit juice	1/2 cup	10	0
Meat, Poultry, Meat Substitutes			
Dried beans, cooked	1/2 cup	44	0
Fish	3 ounces	36	51
Peanut butter	1 tablespoon	11	0
Eggs	1	28	264
Tuna, canned in oil	3 ounces	7	7
Chicken liver	1 ounce	4	160
Beef, pork	3-1/2 ounces	10	70
Luncheon meat	1 ounce	3	22

Table 6.2 (Continued)

Food	Amount	Calcium (mg)	Cholesterol (mg)
	Poor Sources		
Vegetables			
Vegetable	1/2 cup	25	0
Corn	1/2 cup	25	0
Potatoes	1/2 cup	9	0

Sources—Consumer and Food Economics Institute (1976-1980). *Composition of Foods Handbook*. Nos. 8-1, 4, 5, 6, 7. Washington, DC: USDA Agriculture Research Service.

Pennington, J.A.T., & Church, H. (1980). *Food Values of Portions Commonly Used* (13th ed.). New York: Harper & Row.

Robinson, H., & Lawler, M.R. (1982). *Normal and Therapeutic Nutrition* (16th ed.). New York: McMillan.

Schneider, H.A., Anderson, C.E., & Coursin, D.B. (1983). *Nutritional Support of Medical Practice*. (2nd ed). Philadelphia: Harper & Row.

You can estimate your average calcium intake by using Table 6.3, which lists the major food sources of calcium. When completing the checklist, indicate the number of times during the day that you eat any of the items. Then consult the column "Calcium Content of Serving Size Portion" and calculate your calcium intake from each item. To arrive at your total calcium intake for the day, the calcium intakes from all the items should be added together.

The checklist reports intake of calcium from calcium-rich foods only. Smaller amounts of calcium are obtained from other food items as well. The exact amount derived from these items depends on your specific food selections and total caloric consumption but does not generally exceed more than several hundred milligrams. In a diet that excludes dairy products, it is difficult to exceed 300 milligrams of calcium per day. Research using a calcium intake checklist has shown that, by adding a standard factor of 200 milligrams of calcium for foods not included on the checklist, total dietary calcium intake is closely approximated.

HOW TO INCREASE
CALCIUM INTAKE

For the average American woman, increasing daily calcium intake to either 1,000 or 1,500 milligrams calls for significant changes in dietary habits. A quick review of the items listed in the calcium intake checklist (Table 6.3) and the calcium content of foods (Table 6.2) will reveal that most calcium-rich items are dairy products. A 1982 report on the nutritional content of the U.S. food supply indicated that 72% of the available calcium in the American diet came from dairy products. Sardines and salmon that contain the softened bones are also excellent calcium sources. Tofu, or soybean curd, processed with calcium sulfate is an exceptional calcium source. Tofu has been a major source of protein in the Orient for centuries. It is made by solidifying soybeans and water and is usually pressed into squares. Tofu is high in protein but relatively low in fat. Its saturated-fat content is lower than that of chicken, and its cholesterol content is zero. It is used as an ingredient in cooking and can be substituted for meat and cheese in many recipes.

There are several tofu products that are currently sold in supermarkets. To learn to enjoy tofu, you may wish to use it in recipes rather than by itself. Be sure to read the food label when you buy tofu, as the amounts of calcium vary among the different types. For instance, a 4-ounce square of Tomsun's tofu contains almost as much calcium as does a glass of milk. The calcium content of vegetables varies, from sweet corn with almost no calcium to lamb's-quarter with as much as 325 milligrams per serving.

Certain green, leafy vegetables (kale, bok choy, collards, turnip greens, mustard greens, and dandelion greens) also have high calcium content. However, as will be discussed later in this chapter, their oxalic acid content may interfere with the availability of the calcium for absorption. They should not be used as calcium sources. Meat and poultry products are generally poor sources of calcium. An unusual exception is alligator meat, which contains over 1,000 milligrams in a 3-ounce serving. Most cereals are poor sources unless they are enriched, and common fruits and fruit juices are also low in calcium. Nuts vary in their calcium content. Here are several food preparation strategies you might use to increase the calcium content of your diet.

Table 6.3 Calcium Intake Checklist

Food	Serving Size	No. Servings	Calcium Content of Serving Size Portion (mg)	Calculation Column	Calcium Intake (mg)
Milk					
Regular, whole	1 cup	___ cup(s)	291/cup		
2% lowfat	1 cup	___ cup(s)	297/cup		
1% lowfat	1 cup	___ cup(s)	300/cup		
Nonfat, skim	1 cup	___ cup(s)	302/cup		
Chocolate	1 cup	___ cup(s)	287/cup		
Evaporated canned	1 cup	___ cup(s)	657/cup		
Milk beverages					
Eggnog	1 cup	___ cup(s)	330/cup		
Carnation Instant Breakfast	1 cup	___ cup(s)	407/cup		
Milkshake, vanilla	1 cup	___ cup(s)	457/cup		
Thick shake, chocolate	1 cup	___ cup(s)	396/cup		

(Cont.)

Table 6.3 (Continued)

Food	Serving Size	No. Servings	Calcium Content of Serving Size Portion (mg)	Calculation Column	Calcium Intake (mg)
Yogurt					
Plain, unflavored	1 cup	— cup(s)	415/cup		
Fruited	1 cup	— cup(s)	343/cup		
Cheese and cheese products					
American	1 ounce	— ounce(s)	174/ounce		
Blue	1 ounce	— ounce(s)	150/ounce		
Brie/Camembert	1 ounce	— ounce(s)	110/ounce		
Cheddar	1 ounce	— ounce(s)	204/ounce		
Cottage:					
Regular, large curd	1 cup	— cup(s)	135/cup		
Regular, small curd	1 cup	— cup(s)	126/cup		
Lowfat, 2%	1 cup	— cup(s)	155/cup		
Lowfat, 1%	1 cup	— cup(s)	138/cup		
Dry curd cottage	1 cup	— cup(s)	46/cup		
Cream	1 ounce	— ounce(s)	23/ounce		

Mozzarella made with:

Whole milk	1 ounce	___ ounce(s)	163/ounce
Skim milk	1 ounce	___ ounce(s)	207/ounce
Parmesan	1 tablespoon	___ tablespoon(s)	69/tablespoon
Provolone	1 ounce	___ ounce(s)	214/ounce
Ricotta, whole	1 cup	___ cup(s)	509/cup
Ricotta, part skim	1 cup	___ cup(s)	669/cup
Romano cheese	1 ounce	___ ounce(s)	302/ounce
Swiss	1 ounce	___ ounce(s)	272/ounce
Cheese spread, American	1 ounce	___ ounce(s)	159/ounce
Cheez Whiz, Kraft	1 tablespoon	___ tablespoon(s)	75/tablespoon
Cheese sauce, homemade	1 cup	___ cup(s)	89/cup
Other _____		___	

Proteins

Salmon, canned, with bones	1 ounce	___ ounce(s)	55/ounce

(Cont.)

Table 6.3   (Continued)

Food	Serving Size	No. Servings	Calcium Content of Serving Size Portion (mg)	Calculation Column	Calcium Intake (mg)
Proteins					
Sardines, canned	1 ounce	—— ounce(s)	124/ounce		
Shrimp, canned	1 ounce/ 4 medium	—— ounce(s)	33/ounce		
Smelt, canned	4 medium	—— medium	388/medium		
Tofu, soybean curd	1 ounce	—— ounce(s)	35/ounce		
Nuts					
Almonds, chopped	1 cup	—— cup(s)	304/cup		
Almonds, slivered	1 cup	—— cup(s)	269/cup		
Brazil, shelled	1 ounce	—— ounce(s)	53/ounce		
Sesame seed meats	1 cup	—— cup(s)	1,080/cup		
Combination Items					
Cheeseburger	1 ave.	—— ave.	152/ave. serving		

Food	Serving	Calories
Macaroni and cheese (homemade)	1 cup	— cup(s)	362/cup
Macaroni and cheese (box)	1 cup	— cup(s)	199/cup
Pizza, cheese	1/8 12″ pie	— slice	86/slice
Burrito, bean	1 ave.	— ave.	208/ave. serving
Lasagna, Manicotti	1 ave. serving	— ave. serving	252/ave. serving
Cheese soufflé	1 ave. serving	— ave. serving	300/ave. serving
Tostado	1 ave. serving	— ave. serving	191/ave. serving
Desserts			
Custard, baked	1 cup	— cup(s)	297/cup
Frozen yogurt	1 cup	— cup(s)	200/cup
Frozen yogurt bar	1 bar	— bar(s)	78/bar
Ice cream, plain, hard type	1 cup	— cup(s)	176/cup
Ice cream, soft	1 cup	— cup(s)	236/cup
Ice milk	1 cup	— cup(s)	176/cup
Pudding, vanilla	1 cup	— cup(s)	298/cup
Pudding, chocolate	1 cup	— cup(s)	250/cup
Tapioca	1 cup	— cup(s)	173/cup

(Cont.)

Table 6.3 (Continued)

Food	Serving Size	No. Servings	Calcium Content of Serving Size Portion (mg)	Calculation Column	Calcium Intake (mg)
Other					
Broccoli, cooked:					
Stalks, from raw	1 cup	___ cup(s)	136/cup		
Chopped, from frozen	1 cup	___ cup(s)	100/cup		
Waffle, homemade	7" diameter	___ 7" (waffles)	85/waffle		
Waffle, mix	7" diameter	___ 7" (waffles)	179/waffle		
				Calcium intake checklist total = ___	
				Standard calcium intake from other food =	+200
				Total calcium intake =	___

Tips to Increase the Calcium Content of Your Diet

- Add cheese chunks or shredded cheese to salads, vegetables, soups, sandwiches, and meat.
- Use milk (preferably nonfat milk) in cooking whenever possible.
- Add powdered nonfat dry milk to hot beverages and soups and to recipes for cakes, breads, and cookies to enhance calcium content without adding too many calories.
- Add milk or nonfat dry milk to soups.
- Prepare soup stock with the bones of meat and add several teaspoons of vinegar to draw the calcium out of the bones.
- Try tofu (soybean curd) with vegetables, fish or meat.

Remember that by increasing the variety of your food choices, you increase the likelihood that you will be eating a balanced diet.

What About the Fat and Calories in Dairy Products?

A common concern of individuals who must increase their calcium intake is that increasing consumption of dairy products will promote an excessive intake of fat and cholesterol and will result in weight gain and high blood cholesterol. Indeed, when food records of osteoporotic women at the Winthrop-University Hospital Osteoporosis Center were analyzed, it was found that, in an effort to increase the calcium content of their diets, these women did consume more fat and calories than is desirable. To limit fat, cholesterol, and calorie intake but still keep up calcium intake, skim and low-fat varieties of milk, cheese, and yogurt should be used.

For example, all types of milk provide approximately 300 milligrams of calcium per cup, but, due to differences in fat content, their caloric content varies as follows: skim milk 80 calories, 1% low-fat milk 100 calories, 2% low-fat milk 125 calories, and whole milk 160 calories. The cholesterol content of skim milk is only 4 milligrams, low-fat milk is 18 milligrams, and whole milk is 33 milligrams. Water-packed canned salmon, sardines, and tofu are low-fat, low-cholesterol, and low-calorie sources as well. Table 6.2 lists the cholesterol content of various food sources of calcium.

Despite the availability of low-fat dairy products, some women who must closely control their caloric intake find it difficult to achieve the higher recommendations for calcium through the diet alone. This is especially true if one is not fond of milk and yogurt or some of the high-calcium protein sources previously mentioned. The various calorie-level menus (see the appendix to this chapter) were designed by Lynne Sampson-Chimon, MS, RD, to supply 1,500 milligrams of calcium and to approximate the 50% carbohydrate, 20% protein, and 30% fat nutrient distributions recommended for the American diet by the Dietary Guidelines. After looking at the menus it is apparent that, to achieve a 1,500-milligram calcium intake, it is necessary to include a form of dairy product with many of the meals. The lower the calorie level, the more important it is to include a high-calcium food with each meal.

Lactose Intolerance

Another situation in which it is difficult to consume adequate dietary calcium through dairy foods is when an individual is lactose intolerant. This condition is fairly common among blacks and the elderly. The individual has low levels of intestinal lactase, which is an enzyme responsible for breaking down lactose (the primary carbohydrate in milk products) into its simple sugars, namely, glucose and galactose. Symptoms of bloating, gaseousness, and diarrhea are experienced when dairy products are eaten. Individual tolerances to lactose vary greatly. For those with this problem, Lact-Aid, an enzyme preparation that can be added to milk to lower lactose levels, may be helpful in keeping calcium intake up. Low-lactose milk is also available. Yogurt is well tolerated as its bacterial cultures predigest lactose. Cheese may also not present a problem because the molds in cheese remove the lactose. In addition, many individuals have no symptoms if they divide their dairy products evenly among breakfast, lunch, and dinner.

A Look at Calcium-Enriched Foods

The development of calcium-enriched food products by food manufacturers has made it easier for some women to keep up their dietary calcium intake. Recently, each trip to the grocery store seems to reveal a new product that is fortified with calcium. By the beginning of 1987, 25 new calcium-fortified foods were marketed or were being test marketed. There is a low-fat milk with added calcium, and some milk products contain lactaid, a lactase enzyme that aids the digestion of lactose. Manufacturers have also recently released a specially packaged milk that requires no refrigeration and can be stored on the shelf. This is useful for those who wish to bring milk to work or on trips.

There are also light breads with natural calcium and added fiber. Slices of enriched light bread provide approximately 150 milligrams of calcium, whereas a slice of white bread provides only 20. In 1986, General Mills began distributing a calcium-fortified flour. However, the amount of calcium provided is small. Proctor & Gamble produces Citrus Hill Plus Calcium, a fortified juice drink that contains 300 milligrams of calcium per cup with added vitamin D. The Coca-Cola Company is test marketing Tab fortified with 100 milligrams of calcium per can to appeal to its prime market of women 18 to 34 years of age.

A word of caution is needed at this point. Most of the available information about how much calcium is absorbed in the diet comes from studies of foods that are naturally rich in calcium, particularly dairy products. It is not known whether fortified foods will provide a predictable availability of added calcium for absorption and use by the body (bioavailability). For example, a high-fiber grain product could reduce the amount of added calcium that is absorbed. It would be desirable for each fortified product to be tested for the amount of calcium available for absorption. Such studies have been carried out to a limited extent. Until more information is available, do not depend solely on fortified foods for your calcium.

THE U.S. RDA
AND NUTRITION LABELING

The United States Recommended Daily Allowance (U.S. RDA), as distinct from the *RDA* (Recommended Dietary Allowance), is a set of standards developed by the FDA for the purpose of regulating the nutrition labeling of food. The U.S. RDA standard commonly used in nutritional labeling is for adults and children over 4 years. The standard is based on the highest level of a given nutrient in the 1968 RDAs. There are special U.S. RDAs for infants, children under 4 years of age, and pregnant and lactating women. The nutrition label lists the percentage of the U.S. RDA for a variety of vitamins, minerals, and protein provided by a specific portion of the food. The U.S. RDAs are useful for comparing the amounts of different nutrients in different foods.

This labeling program, designed to provide consumers with nutrition information, is voluntary unless a food is enriched or fortified or the food manufacturer makes a nutritional claim. A standard format for the nutrition label has been established (see Figure 6.1). The following information must always be included in the nutrition label: serving size, servings per container, calorie count per serving, protein content per serving in grams, carbohydrate content per serving in grams, fat content per serving in grams, and per serving percentages of the U.S. RDA for protein, vitamin A, vitamin C, thiamine, riboflavin, niacin, calcium, and iron. Other optional nutrients may be included, such as vitamin D, vitamin E, vitamin B_{12}, folic acid, vitamin B_6, phosphorus, iodine, magnesium, zinc, copper, biotin, and pantothenic acid. Fatty-acid composition, cholesterol, and sodium content may also be included.

NUTRITION LABELING

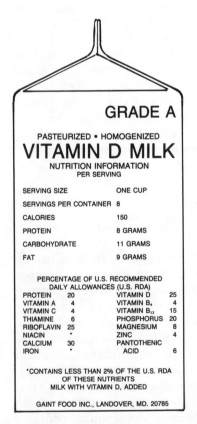

GRADE A   *Grade, if this applies

PASTEURIZED • HOMOGENIZED
VITAMIN D MILK   *Name of Product
NUTRITION INFORMATION
PER SERVING

SERVING SIZE	ONE CUP
SERVINGS PER CONTAINER	8
CALORIES	150
PROTEIN	8 GRAMS
CARBOHYDRATE	11 GRAMS
FAT	9 GRAMS

°Serving Size
°Servings Per Container
°Calories Per Serving
°Protein
°Carbohydrate
°Fat

PERCENTAGE OF U.S. RECOMMENDED
DAILY ALLOWANCES (U.S. RDA)

PROTEIN	20	VITAMIN D	25
VITAMIN A	4	VITAMIN B₄	4
VITAMIN C	4	VITAMIN B₁₂	15
THIAMINE	6	PHOSPHORUS	20
RIBOFLAVIN	25	MAGNESIUM	8
NIACIN	*	ZINC	4
CALCIUM	30	PANTOTHENIC	
IRON	*	ACID	6

*CONTAINS LESS THAN 2% OF THE U.S. RDA
OF THESE NUTRIENTS
MILK WITH VITAMIN D, ADDED

GAINT FOOD INC., LANDOVER, MD. 20785

°Percentage of U.S. RDA for protein and 7 vitamins—Vitamin A, Vitamin C, Thiamine, Riboflavin, Niacin, Calcium, Iron—provided by *one* serving of the product (Any other listings are optional)

Name/Address of Manufacturer or Distributor

Figure 6.1   The information that must appear on labels of all food is indicated with an asterisk (*). Information that must appear on labels of foods that make a nutritional claim is indicated with an open circle (°).

You will recall that the current RDA for calcium is 800 milligrams per day. However, the U.S. RDA for calcium is 1,000 milligrams per day. Therefore, if a label indicates that a product supplies 15% of the U.S. RDA for calcium, then that item provides 150 milligrams of calcium, not 120 as you might calculate using the RDA. It is important to remember that the number of calories and the nutrient information listed on labels are for the serving size specified on the label. When comparing similar food items, you might notice that manufacturers use different serving sizes. This difference will change the nutrient content listings.

Some manufacturers of calcium supplements may list the percentage of U.S. RDA supplied by one or more tablets. For example, a calcium supplement manufacturer states on the label that one tablet provides 60% of the U.S. RDA. Each tablet, therefore, provides 600 milligrams of elemental calcium because 60% of the 1,000 milligrams of the U.S. RDA for calcium is 600 milligrams $(1,000 \times .60 = 600)$.

ACHIEVING AN ADEQUATE CALCIUM INTAKE

The following case demonstrates a strategy that may be used to achieve recommended calcium intake. Sara is a 52-year-old postmenopausal woman who is not taking estrogen. She has been advised to consume 1,500 milligrams of calcium per day. After reviewing the foods listed on the calcium intake checklist, Sara determines that because dairy products are excellent sources of calcium and because she enjoys them, she will emphasize these items in her diet. By including milk (at breakfast, in her tea, at lunch, as an evening snack) and by eating yogurt or ice cream, she can reach a daily calcium intake of 1,225 milligrams. After Sara adds an additional 200 milligrams to account (approximately) for calcium intake from other low-calcium foods in her diet, she estimates that she will be taking in 1,425 milligrams of calcium per day with this new plan. Although her intake is 75 milligrams below the recommended 1,500-milligram level, this small difference is unimportant as on the other days of the week she may consume slightly more than the 1,500 milligrams.

Remember that, when planning dietary calcium intake, it is important to distribute calcium food sources throughout the day as much as possible. Ideally, each meal and snack should contain a high-calcium food. Distributing the intake of calcium throughout the day enhances the total amount of good calcium sources for use at different meals and snack times. A glass of milk for your evening snack may be a good idea.

The Use of Calcium Supplements

Now consider the case of Linda, a 60-year-old postmenopausal woman not taking estrogen who requires 1,500 milligrams of calcium per day and who dislikes milk and yogurt. She is also watching her weight and blood cholesterol level. After reviewing the calcium intake checklist, Linda sees that she likes cheese, ice cream, salmon, and tofu. However, she presently does not eat these items on a daily basis.

Linda decides that, if she has cereal with breakfast daily, she would consume 5 ounces of milk. (With cereal, she can tolerate milk.) Because she is watching her weight and cholesterol intake, she decides to use skim milk. Linda also determines that, if she substitutes water-packed salmon or tofu for other high-fat meats she normally consumes at dinner, she would lower her caloric fat and cholesterol intake and increase her calcium intake. She figures that she could consume 1 cup of tofu (304 milligrams of calcium) or 4 ounces of salmon (220 milligrams of calcium) once each per week.

Because Linda takes her lunch to work, she figures that she can include 2 ounces of low-fat cheese in her diet 5 days per week (250 milligrams of calcium). She plans to do this on days when she does not have tofu or salmon for dinner. She will obtain slightly more than 250 milligrams of calcium per day when the amounts of tofu, salmon, and low-fat cheese are averaged together.

Next, she sees on the calcium and cholesterol content of foods list (Table 6.2) that grated Parmesan cheese has 60 milligrams of calcium per tablespoon. She figures that she can easily add 2 tablespoons of Parmesan cheese to various food items during the day. Linda's daily average calcium intake is 575 milligrams.

Adding the standard 200 milligrams from other dietary calcium sources raises her total calcium intake to 775 milligrams. To meet her calcium needs of 1,500 milligrams, Linda must supplement her diet with approximately 725 milligrams of elemental calcium in the form of a calcium supplement.

Linda plans to take the calcium supplement in the form of three 250-milligram tablets daily. This will provide a total of 1,525 milligrams of elemental calcium, which is slightly more than she needs but is still within an acceptable range.

A Simplified Approach

For those individuals who desire a simplified method of increasing calcium intake the following lists of foods containing 300 and 500 milligrams of calcium will be useful. Use the 300-milligram list or the 500-milligram list, depending on your goal for calcium intake. If your goal is 1,000 milligrams per day, choose one calcium equivalent from the 300-milligram list at each meal. If your goal is 1,500 milligrams per day, use the same strategy using the 500-milligram list. If for some reason you are unable to consume a calcium-equivalent food at any meal, take an equivalent tablet of calcium carbonate. Each evening after dinner, again recall whether you included a calcium-equivalent at each meal. If not, take an equivalent supplement.

These are foods that contain 300 milligrams of calcium:

- Milk, 8 ounces
- Swiss cheese, 1¼ ounces
- Cottage cheese, 2 cups
- Cheddar cheese, 1½ ounces
- Yogurt, fruited, 1 cup
- Ice cream, 1½ cups
- Custard, 1 cup
- Alba Hi-Calcium beverage, 8 ounces
- Homemade macaroni and cheese, ¾ cup
- Tofu, 1 cup
- Almonds, ¾ cup
- Cheese pizza, 2 slices
- Sardines, 6 to 7 medium
- Salmon (canned, with bones), 5 ounces
- Calcium carbonate, 750 milligrams

The following is the list of foods that will provide 500 milligrams of calcium:

- Milk, 14 ounces
- Calcimilk, 8 ounces
- Vanilla milkshake, 12 ounces
- Swiss cheese, 2¼ ounces
- Cottage cheese, 3⅓ cups
- Cheddar cheese, 2½ ounces
- Yogurt, plain, low-fat, 10 ounces
- Ice cream, 2¾ cups

- Custard, 1⅔ cups
- Homemade macaroni and cheese, 1¼ cups
- Tofu, 1¾ cups
- Cheese pizza, 3 slices
- Sardines, 11 medium
- Salmon (canned, with bones), 9 ounces
- Calcium carbonate, 1,250 milligrams

Do not be concerned that your calcium intake is not exact. If your intake is either too low or too high by 200 to 300 milligrams on any given day, it will not make much difference.

OTHER DIETARY FACTORS AND OSTEOPOROSIS

Several dietary factors play important roles in calcium balance. These include vitamin D, lactose, phosphorus and other minerals, protein, sodium, caffeine, fiber, oxalates, phytates, alcohol, vitamins A and C, and any special diets you may follow.

Vitamin D

Recall from chapter 3 that an inadequate vitamin intake is a risk factor for osteoporosis. A hundred years ago 80% of children in the cities of northern and central Europe suffered from rickets, the childhood equivalent of osteomalacia resulting from vitamin D deficiency. The ends of their bones didn't mineralize, and they had reduced growth and bowed legs. Children at that time did not get adequate vitamin D from sunshine. Cod liver oil, which contains vitamin D, was discovered to prevent rickets and was used as a treatment. Although rickets is now rare, mild deficiencies of vitamin D can lead to reduced calcium absorption. The elderly are especially at risk because they may stay indoors, have poorer nutrition, and have an impaired ability to generate calcitriol, the active form of vitamin D. Recently there has been a public education drive to limit exposure to the sun to prevent skin cancer. A few minutes a day in the sun, however, will not increase one's risk for skin cancer. The National Institutes of Health consensus statement on osteoporosis discourages intakes of vitamin D greater than 400 to 800 IU per day. Very large doses (megadoses) of vitamin D cause symptoms such as decreased appetite, nausea, weight loss, intense

thirst, excessive urination, and constipation. A megadose of a vitamin is defined as 10 times the RDA. If blood calcium becomes very
high, life-threatening illness, including coma, may follow. Because
vitamin D is a fat-soluble vitamin, it is stored in the body for a long
period of time, and its toxic effects may persist for several weeks
to months after its use is discontinued.

The American Society for Bone and Mineral Research cautions
that vitamin D intakes in excess of 1,000 IU per day be avoided
unless prescribed by a physician. If a deficiency of vitamin D is suspected, vitamin D levels may be measured in a blood sample. Adequate vitamin D can be obtained by increasing exposure to sunlight
or by dietary modifications that include more foods with vitamin D
such as fortified milk, cheeses, and certain fish. Table 6.4 lists food
sources of vitamin D.

Table 6.4   Food Sources of Vitamin D

Food	Amount	Vitamin D (mg)
Dairy products		
Milk, whole, low-fat, or skim fortified with vitamin D	8 ounces	100
Cheese, Swiss (Emmentaler)	3-1/2 ounces	100
Egg, yolk	1	60
Butter	1 tablespoon	6
Cream, heavy	1 tablespoon	6
Fish		
Eel, smoked	3-1/2 ounces	6,400
Eel, unsmoked	3-1/2 ounces	5,000
Herring	3-1/2 ounces	900
Salmon, Atlantic	3-1/2 ounces	650
Salmon, Atlantic, canned with solids and liquids	3-1/2 ounces	500
Sardines, canned in oil, drained solids	3-1/2 ounces	250
Shrimp, canned, drained solids	3-1/2 ounces	105

(Cont.)

Table 6.4   (Continued)

Food	Amount	Vitamin D (mg)
Mackerel	3-1/2 ounces	50
Oysters	3-1/2 ounces	5
Liver		
Liver, calf or chicken	3-1/2 ounces	50
Oils		
Cod liver oil	1 tablespoon	1,215
Other		
Mushrooms	3-1/2 ounces	150

A multivitamin that provides 400 IU of vitamin D can also serve as a source. When taking calcium supplements that contain vitamin D, be aware of the total vitamin D content so as not to exceed 400 to 800 IU per day. The importance of this practice is supported by the following example. One supplement on the market contains 333 IU of vitamin D and only 89 milligrams of calcium. To obtain 1,000 milligrams of calcium, you would be taking 37,000 IU of vitamin D. Keeping vitamin D intake within the recommended range may mean having two types of calcium supplements on hand, one with vitamin D and one containing only calcium. Another possibility is to take a calcium-only supplement and a multivitamin that provides the RDA for vitamin D.

Lactose

Another nutrient that has been shown to enhance absorption of calcium from the intestine is lactose. It is not known exactly how lactose (more commonly known as "milk sugar") improves calcium absorption.

Phosphorus and Other Minerals

There is little support from studies on humans that phosphorus intake in the range of the average American diet (1,500 to 1,600 milligrams) leads to a deterioration of the calcium balance even though this amount is twice the RDA. Excessive phosphorus intake (i.e., greater than 1,500 milligrams) can be avoided by limiting foods that contain large amounts of phosphorus and small amounts of calcium. Such items include red meats, tuna, soft drinks, and foods with phosphorus additives such as bologna, salami, and other cold cuts as well as bacon and hot dogs.

Fluoride

A fluoride intake of 1.5 to 4.0 milligrams per day for adults is considered safe and may increase calcium retention and decrease bone demineralization as well as reduce the incidence of dental caries. Presently, no evidence justifies exceeding the RDAs of the following metals: zinc (15 milligrams), copper (2 to 3 milligrams), iodine (150 milligrams), manganese (2.5 to 5.0 milligrams), molybdenum (.15 to 0.5 milligrams), selenium (.05 to .06 milligrams), and chromium (.05 to 0.2 milligrams).

Protein

It is generally accepted that the protein content of the American diet is too high. As a result, the 1980 RDAs have a much lower protein recommendation than do the 1968 RDAs. Thus, the current RDA for protein for women 19 years of age and older is 44 grams per day. A more accurate estimation of protein needs is based on the body weight of an individual: 0.8 grams per kilogram of body weight. However, Americans tend to consume twice the RDA, a practice that tends to decrease the kidney's reabsorption of calcium, thereby leading to increased losses of calcium in the urine. It is possible that these losses of calcium in the urine may lead to a negative calcium balance. A person who persists in eating double the recommended amount of protein may increase her calcium requirement by 250 mg per day.

Sodium

Sodium is another nutrient that, when taken in excessive amounts, can cause an increased loss of calcium in the urine. Table salt is 40% sodium and 60% chloride. The average American consumes many times more sodium per day than is needed. Sodium intake in the United States is high due to its heavy use in cooking and at the table and also to its presence in convenience foods. Cutting back on sodium may be healthier for the heart as well as for the bones.

Half the sodium in the American diet is derived from that added in cooking, at the dinner table, and in water. Try to eliminate or reduce added salt.

Caffeine

Excessive caffeine intake can promote loss of calcium through the urine and the stool. Products that contain caffeine include coffee, tea, cola, and chocolate. However, it would take 20 cups of coffee a day to significantly affect calcium balance. The small calcium loss from a few cups of coffee can be easily offset by adding milk.

While excessive protein, sodium, and caffeine may cause an increased loss of calcium through the urine, other dietary factors may interfere with the intestinal absorption of calcium. These are fiber, oxalates, phytates, and alcohol.

Fiber

Because insoluble fibers increase the speed at which the gastro-intestinal tract empties, a very high fiber intake may decrease absorption of dietary calcium. Also, the natural fibers are believed to bind calcium in the intestinal tract. Some studies have suggested that high-fiber diets decrease absorption of calcium from the intestine. However, participants in these studies consumed much higher levels of fiber than is recommended. Fiber has many beneficial attributes, and you should not eliminate it from your diet. Taken in the amounts previously recommended by the Dietary Guidelines, fiber should not affect calcium balance.

Oxalates and Phytates

Oxalates and phytates are substances that bind with calcium in the intestine and make the calcium unavailable to the body. Dark-green, leafy vegetables such as chard, spinach, and collard, beet, and dandelion greens have high calcium contents, but due to the oxalates in these items their calcium is less available. Other foods high in oxalic acid are asparagus, rhubarb, and chocolate. Phytates are found in breads and in cereals such as oatmeal and bran. Because phytates are digested by bacteria in the intestine, it is unlikely that they interfere with calcium absorption. Again, these items should not be eliminated from your diet. However, they should not be counted as good calcium sources either. Presently, it is unclear whether oxalate in one food can combine with the calcium in another food eaten at the same time.

Alcohol

Alcohol is another dietary factor that may interfere with the intestinal absorption of calcium and reduce bone formation. Taken in large enough quantities, alcohol can contribute to a negative calcium balance. Again, there is little evidence that occasional alcohol intake is harmful. However, because excess alcohol reduces bone formation, you cannot overcome its bad effects simply by increasing calcium intake.

Vitamin A

Vitamin A is important for vision, healthy skin, bone growth, reproduction, and the stability of cell membranes. The RDA for vitamin A for nonpregnant and nonlactating women is 800 retinal equivalents or 4,000 IU. Excessive vitamin A (75,000 IU per day) can cause bone loss. Therefore, be cautious when taking vitamin supplements not to overdose on vitamin A.

Vitamin C

Because ascorbic acid (vitamin C) is necessary for the formation of bone matrix, some vitamin enthusiasts have suggested that osteoporotic women take vitamin C supplements. Ascorbic acid levels decline with aging and are reduced in those who smoke cigarettes. However, just as there is little evidence for the many claims made by vitamin enthusiasts, there is no evidence that vitamin C is helpful in preventing or treating osteoporosis. Indeed, there is reason to believe that megadoses of vitamin C promote bone loss. Unless new studies show otherwise, only 50 to 100 milligrams of vitamin C should be obtained daily through either diet or a supplement.

VEGETARIAN AND WEIGHT-LOSS DIETS

Americans vary in their attitudes and behaviors toward food. They also vary in their care in selecting their diets. This section discusses several popular current diet choices.

Vegetarian Diets

Many Americans today are eating vegetarian diets. From the standpoint of calcium balance, a vegetarian diet can be healthy as long as an adequate amount of food is consumed. The dark-green, leafy vegetables mentioned previously that contain oxalates should not be depended on as calcium sources. Individuals on strict "vegan" diets, which eliminate all meats, fish, poultry, eggs, and dairy products, obtain very little calcium and other nutrients. A registered dietitian should be consulted for recommendations about special food products and vitamin and mineral supplements that can be used to increase calcium and other nutrient consumption.

Weight-Loss Diets

The United States is a weight-conscious society. This is reflected by the multibillion-dollar diet industry that exists in this country today. We often resort to fad diets or extremely low calorie diets to promote weight loss. These diets are almost always low in calcium, and their prolonged or repeated use can leach calcium from the bones, thus increasing the chances of developing osteoporosis later in life. When dieting, follow a well-balanced diet that is supplemented with calcium as needed. For women who exercise vigorously it is essential to increase caloric intake to avoid amenorrhea and estrogen deficiency.

Nutritional Myths and Quackery

The current popular interest in nutrition has many advantages. Many individuals are now consuming a healthier diet than they were in the past. However, there are some who capitalize on this interest by promoting nutritional "information" that has no scientific basis and that may claim to cure illnesses that "ordinary" physicians are unable to cure. They also claim that they are suppressed by the FDA, the AMA, and the "medical establishment." Beware of individuals who push large doses of vitamins or foods with "magical powers." They want you to believe that there is an easy way to solve weight or medical problems. For accurate nutrition information, a registered dietitian should be consulted. You may find a registered dietitian by contacting your local hospital, a physician, or a local dietetic association.

SUMMARY

This chapter presented you with dietary guidelines for building and maintaining a healthy skeleton as well as recommendations for preventing osteoporosis. The estrogen-deficient woman may require as much as 1,500 milligrams of calcium per day, and premenopausal women need 1,000 milligrams. Increasing calcium intake is not as effective as taking estrogen in preventing bone loss. It is best to obtain calcium from food sources rather than supplements. If you find this difficult due to food preferences or intolerances, a calcium supplement may be more convenient. In the elderly, a vitamin D supplement of 400 IU may be helpful.

Another dietary approach you can take to prevent osteoporosis is to limit your consumption of the substances that either promote the loss of calcium from the body or interfere with the absorption of calcium from the intestines. This means avoiding excessive intakes of phosphorous, protein, sodium, caffeine, fiber, alcohol, and megadoses of vitamins and minerals. You need to carefully plan low-calorie and vegetarian diets to ensure that you are getting an adequate nutritional balance.

APPENDIX

Daily Menus for 1,200-, 1,500-, 1,800-Calorie/ 1,500-Milligram Calcium Diets

DAILY MENUS FOR A 1,200-CALORIE/1,500-MILLIGRAM DIET

Breakfast

- ¼ cup Farina, dry
- 1 tablespoon diet margarine
- ½ cup orange juice
- 1 cup skim milk

Lunch

- 1 cup tomato soup made with skim milk
- 1 slice whole wheat bread
- 1 ounce diet cheese (e.g., Weight Watcher's)
- 1 tablespoon diet margarine

Dinner

- 3 ounces tomato surprise with canned salmon
- 3 Ry-Krisp crackers
- 1 cup green beans
- 1 tablespoon diet margarine
- 1 cup iced tea

Snack

- 8 ounces plain low-fat yogurt
- ½ sliced banana
- 1 teaspoon sugar (or artificial sweetener)

Total Calcium = 1,572 mg

Breakfast

- ½ grapefruit
- 1 ounce diet cheese
- 1 slice whole wheat bread
- 1 cup skim milk
- 1 teaspoon margarine

Lunch

- Chef's salad:
  1 cup raw spinach
  1 medium tomato
  ¼ cup celery
  1 ounce diet cheese
- 3 Ry-Krisp crackers
- 2 teaspoons oil
- 1 teaspoon vinegar
- ½ cup any fresh fruit
- ½ cup skim milk

Dinner

- 3 ounces roast turkey
- 1 cup mashed potato
- ½ cup string beans
- 1 rounded teaspoon cranberry sauce
- 1 teaspoon margarine
- ½ cup any fresh fruit
- 1 cup skim milk

Snack

- ½ cup low-calorie pudding made with skim milk

Total Calcium = 1,589 mg

Breakfast

- ¾ cup blueberries
- 8 ounces plain low-fat yogurt
- 1 slice whole wheat bread
- 1 teaspoon margarine

Lunch

- Vegetable pita:
  ½ cup 2% cottage cheese mixed with 2 teaspoons nonfat powdered milk
  1 tablespoon Parmesan cheese
  1/8 cup green pepper
  2 small radishes
  1 small tomato
  1 pita bread
  ½ teaspoon Italian dressing
- 1 small orange
- ½ cup skim milk

Dinner

- Broccoli-cheese stuffed potato:
  1 medium potato
  ½ cup broccoli spears
  2 slices diet cheese
- Lettuce wedge
- 2 teaspoons oil
- 1 teaspoon vinegar

Snack

- Frozen banana shake:
  ½ medium banana
  ½ cup skim milk
  Noncaloric sweetener
- Dash nutmeg

Total Calcium = 1,503 mg

DAILY MENUS FOR A 1,500-CALORIE/1,500-MILLIGRAM CALCIUM DIET

Breakfast

- ¾ cup blueberries
- 8 ounces plain low-fat yogurt
- 1 slice whole wheat bread
- 1 teaspoon margarine

Lunch

- 1 cup tomato soup made with skim milk and additional 2 table-spoons instant nonfat dry milk
- Tossed salad:
  Lettuce
  Small tomato
  ½ large carrot
  2 ounces tofu
  1 tablespoon Parmesan cheese
  2 teaspoons oil
  1 teaspoon vinegar
- 6 saltines
- ½ cup any fresh fruit

Dinner

- 3 ounces canned salmon patty with ¼ cup cheese sauce
- ½ cup peas
- ½ cup rice
- 1 teaspoon margarine
- ½ cup any fresh or canned fruit

Snack

- ½ cup vanilla pudding made with whole milk

Total Calcium = 1,496 mg

Breakfast

- ½ cup grapefruit juice
- 1 whole wheat English muffin
- 1 teaspoon margarine
- 8 ounces skim milk

Lunch

- 2 ounces low-fat Swiss cheese
- 1 large carrot
- 2 slices whole wheat bread
- ½ cup fresh fruit
- 4 ounces skim milk
- 1 teaspoon margarine

Dinner

- 4 ounces broiled chicken
- ½ cup broccoli
- Medium baked potato
- Small pear
- 1 teaspoon margarine
- 4 ounces skim milk

Snack

- 1 cup vanilla ice cream

Total Calcium = 1,532 mg

Breakfast

- 1 cup Shredded Wheat cereal
- 4 ounces 1% low-fat milk
- 1 egg
- 1 slice wheat toast
- 1 teaspoon margarine
- 1 teaspoon jelly
- 4 ounces orange juice
- Coffee, black

Lunch

- Sandwich:
  2 slices white bread
  2 ounces American cheese
  1 teaspoon mustard
- 1 orange
- 8 ounces 1% low-fat milk

Snack

- ¼ cup almonds

Dinner

- 3 ounces broiled fish
- 1 baked potato
- 2 teaspoons margarine

- 1 cup broccoli
- 1 small roll (plain)
- ¼ cantaloupe
- Iced tea

Total Calcium = 1,500 mg

DAILY MENUS FOR A 1,800-CALORIE/1,500-MILLIGRAM CALCIUM DIET

Breakfast

- 1 cup orange juice
- 1 whole wheat English muffin
- 1 ounce melted Swiss cheese
- ½ cup fresh fruit

Lunch

- 2 ounces roast turkey
- 2 slices whole wheat bread
- 2 teaspoons mayonnaise
- Lettuce
- 1 large or several small raw carrot sticks
- 8 ounces part skim plain yogurt
- ½ cup fresh fruit

Dinner

- 3 ounces broiled chicken
- ½ cup broccoli
- 1 medium baked potato topped with ½ ounce cheddar cheese
- 8 ounces skim milk
- 1 tablespoon mayonnaise
- ½ cup fresh fruit

Snack

- ½ cup fresh fruit
- 1 cup vanilla ice cream

Total Calcium = 1,543 mg

7 CHAPTER

The Estrogen Controversy

Between 10,000 B.C. and A.D. 1640, the life span of women increased by only 4 years, from age 28 to 32. Not until 1800 did the life span reach the current age of menopause (around 51). Today, women who reach the average age of menopause can expect to live 30 more years. This means that the modern woman lives more than one third of her life after menopause. The transition from the reproductive stage of life to old age is often referred to as the *climacteric*.

Menopause is caused by aging of the ovaries and the resulting loss of the ovarian hormones, estrogens and progestins. A lack of these hormones results in the end of menstruation and in problems associated with menopause, for example, vaginal dryness, hot flushes, urinary symptoms, depression, and osteoporosis. Replacing these hormones in the form of medication alleviates all these problems. In addition, estrogens may be protective against heart disease.

WHAT IS THE ESTROGEN CONTROVERSY?

Why aren't all postmenopausal women placed on estrogen therapy? This can best be explained by describing a problem the Winthrop-University Hospital research group encountered when we planned a research study over a decade ago concerning the effect of estrogens on postmenopausal bone loss.

Our first problem was finding women to participate in the study; most volunteers on Long Island were already taking estrogen. The practice of the day was estrogen therapy at the first hot flash— "feminine forever" was the slogan of the 1960s and early 1970s.

After we succeeded in enrolling a number of women in our study, the media publicized results from a study that linked taking estrogen with an increased incidence of endometrial cancer (cancer of the lining of the uterus). The publicity led to an estrogen "scare" equivalent to the calcium craze in magnitude. A number of women in our study refused to continue to participate. We decided to take a biopsy of the *endometrium* (the lining of the uterus) of each participant prior to administering estrogen. What had once been a routine process of administering estrogen had been transformed into a complicated process requiring careful medical supervision. Because of the cancer scare among women in the study, we decided to discontinue the project.

Fortunately, other researchers managed to complete similar studies, which clearly showed that estrogen therapy prevented the bone loss that occurs after the ovaries are removed or after natural menopause. When researchers compared fracture patients with women of the same age with no fractures, they discovered that estrogen administration protected against fractures of the hip, spine, and wrist. There is absolutely no question about the effectiveness of estrogens in preventing postmenopausal bone loss. In April 1986, the FDA finally approved the use of estrogen as effective in preventing postmenopausal bone loss and in treating osteoporosis. This chapter discusses the benefits and risks of hormonal replacement therapy and describes aggressive and conservative approaches to the management of menopause.

THE BENEFITS OF ESTROGEN TREATMENT

Menopausal problems other than bone loss respond to estrogen therapy, such as vulvogenital atrophy and *vasomotor flushes* (hot flashes). The *vulva, vagina, urethra,* and *bladder trigone* are related in embryologic development, and all are estrogen responsive. Following menopause, there is *atrophy* of these tissues, and the following symptoms may be troublesome: vaginal dryness, pain during intercourse, vaginal burning, increased urinary frequency, and pain on urination in the absence of urinary tract infection. Oral and topical (locally applied) estrogens relieve these symptoms. The estrogen deficiency results in a decreased blood supply to the tissues and a decrease in vaginal lubrication. These conditions are usually treated intermittently; that is, there is a course of treatment, the symptoms vanish, and treatment is readministered when the symptoms recur.

Effective Treatment of Hot Flashes

Vasomotor flushes trouble three quarters of women of menopausal age. These flushes give the sensation of heat and are accompanied by sweating. Estrogen is the most effective drug for preventing flushes. Usually, it can be given for a short period of time, but 20% of women continue to have flushes for 5 years after menopause.

Effective Treatment of Insomnia

In the past, *involutional melancholia* (a specific depressive illness) was attributed to menopause. The existence of emotional illness related to estrogen deficiency has not been documented. However, insomnia is clearly associated with menopause. Recently, sleep centers have studied night awakening in menopausal women that occurs with hot flashes. When women are given estrogens, the flashes diminish and sleep improves.

Estrogen deficiency possibly produces a *sleep deprivation syndrome*. This term applies to symptoms resulting from a lack of sleep. Anyone who has been denied sleep for a prolonged time is familiar with the resulting fatigue, irritability, and difficulty with concentration. The relief from insomnia may be the reason why estrogens produce a general feeling of well-being in some women.

Protection Against Atherosclerosis

It has been known for a long time that, until menopause, women have less coronary artery disease than do men. A large-scale study of men who had survived heart attacks failed to show a benefit of estrogen administration, and this led to a decline in interest concerning a protective effect of estrogen against atherosclerosis (hardening of the arteries). However, it is apparent that estrogen should not be expected to have the same effects in men as in women.

Interest has rekindled recently in estrogen's possible protective effect against atherosclerosis. Estrogens have been shown to increase blood levels of HDL (high-density lipoproteins), which are believed to remove cholesterol and to protect against atherosclerosis. Several studies using a case-control method (performed by comparing patients with a disease with those who do not have the disease) have yielded conflicting results. One study found a seven-fold increase in heart attacks in users of estrogens from 39 to 45 years of age (Jick, Dinian, & Rothman, 1978). However, all but one of the victims of *myocardial infarction* were cigarette smokers (cigarette smoking is, of course, a powerful risk factor for heart attack). A recent case-control study of American nurses supported a protective effect of estrogens (Bain et al., 1981) against myocardial infarction.

A similar study in a Los Angeles retirement community showed that women who were not given estrogens had 2.3 times the number of heart attacks compared to those who took estrogens (Ross, Paganini-Hill, & Mack, 1981). More research is required to show that estrogens are definitely protective against heart attack in post-menopausal women, although there is a growing appreciation that this may become the most important reason for women to take estrogens. Indeed, because heart attack is a major killer, if estrogen replacement therapy prevents heart attack, it is likely that discussion about estrogen for the prevention of osteoporosis will diminish and we will reenter the stage of "feminine forever."

THE POTENTIAL RISKS OF ESTROGEN TREATMENT

In addition to endometrial cancer, the potential risks of estrogen-replacement therapy include hypertension, gallbladder disease, and abnormal uterine bleeding. Breast cancer as a risk remains controversial, but the latest evidence suggests that estrogen use does not cause breast cancer. There is no clear evidence of adverse effects of estrogen-replacement therapy on psychiatric disorders, heart attack, stroke, *pulmonary embolism*, and diabetes.

In July 1977, the commissioner of the FDA issued a new warning to be included in the package inserts for all estrogens. Because of the controversy concerning the safety of estrogens, a National Institutes of Health consensus-development conference, "Estrogen and Women," was held. In 1983, the Council of Scientific Affairs of the AMA published a report for the public and the practicing physician. The council's findings concerning the risk of estrogens will be repeated here.

The AMA Risk Report and Other Studies

The council reported that the incidence of endometrial cancer in postmenopausal women not treated with estrogen is about 1 case per 1,000 women per year (0.1%). Three case-control studies found an increased risk of endometrial cancer from estrogen use. Case-control studies are performed by comparing patients with a disease with similar patients who do not have the disease. Interpretation of such studies is hazardous unless the two groups of patients are comparable for all the factors that influence whether they are at risk for the disease in question. These studies found that the risk of developing endometrial cancer was increased two to eight times when estrogens were used daily for 2 to 4 years and that the risk declined when estrogen use ceased. An increased risk was questionable in women with other predisposing factors such as obesity and *nulliparity* (never having been pregnant). If the findings of these studies are valid, then the increased risk would result in a 0.2% to 0.8% annual incidence of endometrial cancer in estrogen users. There would be two to eight new cases of endometrial cancer each year for every 1,000 women taking estrogen.

Other studies have concluded that there is no relationship between estrogen use and endometrial cancer. One of these studies was prospective. A prospective study concerning estrogen and endometrial cancer involves monitoring two groups for the development of endometrial cancer—one group takes estrogen, and the other does not. Prospective studies are viewed more favorably by scientists because they do not have the same methodological problems that case-control studies have. Nonetheless, the council cautiously concluded that estrogen administration increases the incidence of endometrial cancer. The conclusion was based on the following evidence:

- Animal experiments suggest that estrogens increase cancer in other tissues.
- The risk of cancer in the case-control studies increased with higher doses of estrogens and length of use.
- The evidence of endometrial cancer increased in particular regions of the United States in parallel with an increased national use of estrogens. As a result of subsequent studies, there is general agreement that estrogens increase the risk of endometrial cancer.

In cases of endometrial cancer that arise from estrogen use, the cancer behaves in a less aggressive manner. Thus, 5-year survival rates for endometrial cancer in those who take estrogen have been reported to be 90% to 95%. (The mortality rates from cancer are usually given as the percentage of patients living 5 years after diagnosis; for many types of cancer, the 5-year survival rate is only about 20%.) In addition, although there was an increase in the number of new cases of endometrial cancer in parallel with increased estrogen use in the United States, there was no increase in regional or national deaths from this disease. This led to the second conclusion of the council: Although estrogen increases the number of cases of uterine cancer, it does not increase the death rate from this disease. The council also came to the conclusion that adding progestin to the *cyclic* administration of estrogen (estrogen for 21 to 25 days of the month) probably results in a lower incidence of endometrial cancer.

AMA Council Recommendations

The council also reviewed evidence for other adverse effects of estrogen and noted that most such claims were based on studies of young women using oral contraceptives. Thus, the evidence was not applicable to older women using lower doses of estrogen. The adverse effects include gallbladder disease, *benign* liver tumors, high blood pressure, and high blood glucose. It also concluded that "studies attempting to identify a possible relationship between menopausal estrogen therapy and breast cancer have not produced significant evidence of such a link" (Council on Scientific Affairs, 1983).

The council report concluded with eight recommendations for the management of menopause:

- Estrogens should be used only for purposes that respond to estrogens and in the smallest effective dose for the shortest period possible.
- Estrogens are effective in the treatment or prevention of hot flashes, menopausal *urogenital* symptoms, and osteoporosis. They may protect against heart disease.
- When estrogens are given to a woman who has not had a hysterectomy, the estrogen should be given in a cycle (21 days of the month); a progestin may be given on the last 7 to 10 days of the cycle.
- Vaginal cream may be useful for local urogenital disease.
- Vaginal bleeding between cycles should be promptly investigated.
- Patients on estrogens must be evaluated yearly, have their blood pressure taken, and have breast and pelvic (internal) exams. *Histologic* and *cytologic* sampling of the cervix and uterus may be included in the pelvic exam.
- Estrogen should not be given to anyone with known cancer or a history of breast cancer.
- The patient should be fully informed of risks and benefits of estrogen use. Discontinuation of estrogen should be considered periodically.

An important point that should be made concerning the estrogen controversy refers to the council's first recommendation, that estrogens be given "for the shortest period necessary." Unlike other reasons for using estrogen-replacement therapy, the prevention of osteoporosis implies prolonged estrogen use. When estrogens are discontinued in postmenopausal women after several years, rapid bone loss follows, just as it would if estrogens were not given at menopause. Thus, estrogen use only delays the bone loss after menopause for as long as the estrogen is taken. Unfortunately, the risk of side effects such as endometrial cancer increases with the length of estrogen use. It is not known how long estrogens must be taken to prevent osteoporosis, but most physicians would prescribe them until about age 65.

MEDICATIONS USED IN ESTROGEN-REPLACEMENT THERAPY

The term estrogen does not refer to a specific hormone that is made by the ovaries. Rather, the term is used to describe many compounds, some natural (made by the ovaries), some synthetic (created in the laboratory), and some natural but produced by tissues other than the ovaries. Estrogen is defined as a compound having two biological effects: (a) the ability to stimulate specific changes in the genital organs and (b) the ability to maintain secondary sexual characteristics (the changes that occur in women after puberty). Diverse chemical compounds have these biological effects. Therefore, it is not surprising that estrogenic compounds may differ in their effects on organs (such as the liver) and may have side effects. The commonly prescribed compounds are presented in Table 7.1.

There are three natural estrogens: estrone, estradiol, and estriol. These hormones are synthesized from other hormones that are considered to be androgens (masculinizing hormones). The most commonly prescribed estrogens are the three natural ones, products derived from them, and the synthetic compounds ethinyl estradiol and mestranol. The minimum effective dose to prevent postmenopausal bone loss is 0.625 milligrams of *conjugated estrogens* or its equivalent. One recent study (Ettinger, Genant, & Cann, 1987) suggests that a lower dose of estrogen may suffice when diet is supplemented with calcium.

Because many of the adverse effects of estrogens may result from their metabolism by the liver following absorption, other routes for

Table 7.1 Estrogen Preparations

Generic	Lowest effective daily dose (mg)[a]	Trade name
Conjugated	0.3 to 0.625	Premarin
Ethinyl estradiol	0.01 to 0.02	Estinone
		Feminone
Micronized estradiol	1.0	Estrace
Diethylstilbesterol (DES)	0.2	Diethylstilbesterol
Quinestrol	0.1	Estrovis
Piperazine estrone sulfate	0.625	Ogen
Esterified estrogens	0.3	Amnestrogen
		Evex
		Menest
		Estratab
Combined estrogens	1 tablet	Hormonin
Transdermal estradiol		Estraderm

[a]Doses are effective for many of the symptoms of estrogen deprivation. The lowest dose for the prevention of postmenopausal bone loss is 0.625 milligrams or its equivalent of conjugated estrogens.

estrogen administration have been sought. One technique is to apply estrogen to the skin. Absorption of estrogen through the skin *(transdermal)* bypasses the liver and theoretically would avoid some undesirable effects. Transdermal systems of medication delivery have been used for *nitroglycerine* in the treatment of heart disease and for scopolamine for motion sickness. The FDA approved the use of a transdermal system for estradiol in 1986. The patch is transparent and is applied to the skin twice weekly, and it may be worn while swimming or bathing. Transdermal estradiol delivers blood levels of estrogens similar to those occurring in premenopausal women and does not raise blood pressure. The FDA will probably approve transdermal estrogens for prevention and treatment of osteoporosis after studies are completed that demonstrate that they are as effective as oral estrogens. There is no reason to believe that this will not be the case as studies conducted in Europe have already shown that transdermal estrogens prevent bone loss.

THE ROLE OF PROGESTINS IN ESTROGEN-REPLACEMENT THERAPY

Progestational agents, or progestins (compounds with effects like progesterone), may be given in combination with estrogen. During the menstrual cycle, progesterone is manufactured after ovulation. Progesterone modulates the effect of estrogen on tissues in a variety of complex ways. Not only is progesterone withdrawal responsible for menstruation, but progesterone levels influence the effects of estrogens on enzymes and the ability of estrogen to bind to the cells it affects.

The forerunner of cancer of the uterus is *endometrial hyperplasia* (an excess number of cells of the uterine lining). Many of the risk factors for the development of endometrial cancer seem to be related to the long-term unopposed effects of estrogen. Thus, an increased risk of endometrial cancer is higher with continuous rather than cyclic estrogen administration (21 to 25 days of the month).

Several studies have examined the incidence of endometrial cancer in untreated patients compared with those treated with estrogen alone and estrogen combined with progestins. Those who receive progestins appear to be better protected against endometrial cancer than do the untreated groups (MacDonald, 1981). Almost all the patients who received progestins and yet developed endometrial cancer took progestins only 5 to 7 days of the month. Thus, it has been recommended that a progestin should be given for 10 to 13 days of the month to simulate the menstrual cycle more closely. Some studies suggest that as low a dose as 2.5 milligrams of medroxyprogesterone acetate (one of the commonly used progestins) may be effective. However, further studies must be performed before the lower dose can be recommended.

In a recent study from King's College and the Chelsea Hospital in London (Padwick, Pryse-Davies, & Whitehead, 1986), it was suggested that the dose of progestin should be adjusted so that regular menstrual bleeding occurs on or after day 11 after starting the progestin. When this is done, there appears to be no need for endometrial biopsy.

Progestins probably have a bone-sparing effect similar to that of estrogens. Indeed, if estrogens cannot be used for replacement therapy, progestins are sometimes substituted. In addition, it is believed that progestins counterbalance the effect of estrogens on the breast and may be protective against the development of breast cancer. Some physicians advocate the use of progestins whenever estrogen is given to prevent breast cancer. A positive relationship between estrogen and breast cancer remains unproven, so there is no known value in women taking progestins if they have had a hysterectomy (without a uterus, women are obviously not at risk for endometrial hyperplasia or uterine cancer).

Furthermore, some physicians prefer not to use progestins in all women. They point out (and correctly) that there is little information concerning the long-term risks of combined estrogen-progestin treatment of postmenopausal women. In younger women who take oral contraceptives (at higher doses of both estrogen and progestin), there is an increased risk of pulmonary embolism, heart attack, and stroke. In addition, some progestins may lower HDL levels so that there is a theoretic consideration that they may counteract the beneficial effect of estrogens in preventing heart disease. Progestins may produce symptoms that resemble premenstrual tension syndrome: depression, bloating, cramps, pelvic pressure, and fluid retention. Until the long-term risks of progestins in postmenopausal women are known, some physicians are reserving progestins only for women on estrogen-replacement therapy who develop endometrial hyperplasia and uterine bleeding. Of course, if estrogens are given alone, endometrial biopsy must still be performed.

Some physicians administer a progestin for each day that estrogen is given so the estrogen and a progestin are taken from the first through the 25th day of each month. The advantage of this regimen is that 90% of women do not have uterine bleeding. If bleeding occurs, then both hormones are given continuously through the month. Although this regimen should protect against endometrial cancer and has the advantage of preventing uterine bleeding, further studies need to be done before it can be generally recommended.

AGGRESSIVE VERSUS CONSERVATIVE MENOPAUSE MANAGEMENT

Now that the risks and benefits of hormone replacement therapy at menopause are better understood, let us consider different approaches to the management of menopause. The recommendations given by the Council of Scientific Affairs and other groups represent consensus opinions and are appropriately conservative. An increasing number of physicians, however, believe that we should be more aggressive in the management of menopause in every woman. In concluding this chapter, two approaches will be presented: an aggressive approach and a more conservative approach. It is apparent that the estrogen scare, caused in part by media attention, has almost ended. Indeed, it is being replaced by an osteoporosis scare. Most authorities have not returned full cycle to the "feminine-forever" era. Nonetheless, everyone agrees that, if proper selection is used, women should not be denied the advantages of estrogen-replacement therapy. In the remainder of this chapter, the different philosophical approaches to menopause will be discussed and the estrogen controversy placed in perspective.

The Aggressive Approach

Abundant sexist references in English literature exist that concern women living beyond their "useful" reproductive years. The atrophy of an endocrine organ in adult life occurs only in the ovary. Atrophy of any other endocrine organ is called a "disease," whereas atrophy of the ovary is called "natural" because it occurs in all women.

Atrophy of the testes (male *gonads*) is called *hypogonadism*. Male hypogonadism is associated with osteoporosis. There is absolutely no controversy over giving hypogonadal men testosterone (the masculinizing hormone that is the male counterpart of estrogens) or synthetic masculinizing hormones. Why, then, is there such concern in women? One reason is the hesitation by scientists to make

recommendations for large populations. Incorrect recommendations could affect the female population of the entire world. In addition, the technology available in the United States, such as an
endometrial biopsy, is too expensive for undeveloped countries.

A more progressive approach begins with the idea that women
in developed countries should not suffer because scientists are unwilling to make global recommendations and that menopause is a
hormonal deficiency disorder that should be corrected by hormonal
replacement therapy with the guidance of a physician. Progestins
are given cyclically in the perimenopausal period, when women
may have irregular periods. Eventually, the progestins no longer
produce withdrawal bleeding, indicating that estrogen levels are
low. A blood estrogen level is obtained to confirm this, and a base-
line *mammogram* is performed. An endometrial as well as cervi-
cal sample is obtained, and estrogen is added to the replacement
regimen (progestins are continued). The diet is adjusted to include
1,000 to 1,200 milligrams of calcium per day and 400 IU of vitamin D. An assessment of physical activity is made, and the woman
is encouraged to participate in an exercise program. The estrogens
and progestin are continued indefinitely. The usual replacement
therapy is the equivalent of 0.625 milligrams of conjugated combined estrogen for 25 days of the month and 5 to 10 milligrams of
medroxyprogesterone acetate for 11 to 25 days of the month.

For women with absolute contraindications to estrogen use,
progesterone is used instead, and, if needed, calcium supplements
are given to achieve a daily intake of 1,500 milligrams per day.
Enthusiasts for "feminine forever" point out that not only will osteoporosis and urogenital atrophy be prevented but also that atrophy
of the skin will be prevented and a feeling of well-being will ensue.
The risk of women taking estrogens dying from endometrial cancer
if periodic cytologic samplings are taken is probably less than that
in women who have never taken estrogens and who are not carefully followed by a gynecologist. There is no increased risk of
developing endometrial cancer if progestins are added to the estrogen therapy.

The Conservative Approach

The evaluation of menopausal women by mammography and endometrial sampling and the addition of progestins is the same
whether a physician recommends an aggressive or a conservative

approach. The major difference in the two schools of thought is that the conservative school will treat only 20% to 30% of women with estrogen for a prolonged period of time, whereas the aggressive school will treat almost all women for their entire life spans after menopause.

Current estrogen-replacement therapy is imperfect and does not exactly replicate the hormonal milieu prior to menopause. A major difficulty in accomplishing this concerns the chemical character- istics of estrogens. Chemical modifications are necessary for the estrogen compounds to be absorbed consistently from the gastro- intestinal tract or for long-acting preparations to be effective when injected into muscle. Moreover, the blood vessels from the gastro- intestinal tract drain into the liver, where estrogens are chemically modified. The ovaries secrete estrogen directly into the circulation, which carries the estrogen to its target tissues. Unfortunately, the liver changes the absorbed estrogens into different compounds. Many believe that a number of side effects of estrogen are due to the changes that occur as it passes through the liver.

The development of a transdermal system for estrogen was a major breakthrough toward optimal estrogen therapy. This form of estrogen therapy should convert even the most conservative phy- sician to recommend estrogen use more frequently. However, mem- bers of the conservative school insist that further studies with the transdermal estrogen systems must be completed and that the long- term effects of progestins need more study.

What are the specific indications for estrogen use? Hot flashes are treated until they decrease to a tolerable level. This usually oc- curs in several months, but an unusual case may require treatment for 2 to 5 years. Urogenital complaints are treated with a vaginal estrogen cream; only if this is unsuccessful is oral or transdermal estrogen given. If the symptoms subside in 6 months to 1 year, the estrogens are discontinued.

Because only 20% to 25% of women develop osteoporotic frac- tures, only roughly this number of postmenopausal women should be selected for lifetime estrogen use. Selection is based on identify- ing those women who are at high risk for osteoporosis in the future. Members of the conservative school also emphasize that gynecologi- cal problems increase with estrogen use. Women who take estrogen have vaginal bleeding five times as often as women who do not and, as a result, undergo *D & Cs* (dilatation and curettage) for diagnosis six times as often. They have hysterectomies seven times as often as women who do not take estrogen.

SUGGESTIONS FOR RECOMMENDING TREATMENT OPTIONS

Often, after I explain to a patient all the risks and benefits of treatment or a procedure, I am asked, "But what do you recommend, doctor?" First, the only way the decision should be made is by an informed patient with the advice of a physician who is thoroughly familiar with her state of health and with the risk of her using estrogens.

American women have generally decided against prolonged estrogen use. There are 40 million women in the United States who are estrogen deficient, and only 4 to 5 million of them take estrogens! I believe that one reason for this is the reluctance of women to accept having periods (vaginal bleeding) in mid-life and later. Indeed, new methods of hormonal replacement therapy that avoid vaginal bleeding are currently being investigated.

In 1986, a study was published (Hillner, Hollenberg, & Pauker, 1986) that evaluated the risks and benefits of estrogen-replacement therapy in light of current knowledge. This study considered the multiple possible outcomes of taking or not taking estrogen. The authors concluded that the benefits of taking estrogen outweigh the risks. Most important, the authors emphasized that, if it is proven that estrogen is protective against developing coronary artery disease, this protective effect overwhelmingly makes estrogen-replacement therapy beneficial (with little risk) for most women. Benefits outweigh risks even if there were no effect on the heart. If research in the next 5 to 10 years establishes a protective effect on heart disease, "feminine forever" will be back in vogue. One unanswered question, however, concerns the effects of progestins. It is not known whether adding progestins will adversely influence the beneficial effects of estrogen. It is possible, for example, that the protective effect of estrogen against heart disease will not persist if certain progestins are also given. The facts about hormonal replacement therapy are listed below.

- Estrogen prevents postmenopausal bone loss.
- Estrogen (given alone) increases the risk of endometrial cancer.
- Estrogen probably protects women against coronary artery disease.
- Estrogen does not increase the risk of breast cancer.
- Progestins (added to estrogen therapy) protect against endometrial cancer.
- It is not known whether adding certain progestins reduces the protective effect of estrogens on coronary artery disease.

At present I place only women who are at high risk for osteoporosis on prolonged estrogen therapy. If there are major risks of estrogen use present in the woman, estrogens should not be used. Estrogens should not be taken if you have active liver disease, if your mother or sister had breast cancer, or if you had a breast biopsy that was suspicious. Be cautious in using estrogens if you have high blood pressure or gallbladder disease; transdermal estrogens may be preferable in these instances. Adequate calcium, exercise, and health promotion is advised for all menopausal women.

If there are no contraindications, the woman is placed on estrogen following a negative mammogram (no evidence of breast cancer), Pap test of the cervix, and in some cases endometrial sampling by her gynecologist. For the present, I would continue estrogen until about the age of 65, prolonging the climacteric for about 15 years.

Until more information is available, progestins are recommended for the last 14 days of the cycle in addition to the equivalent of 0.625 milligrams of conjugated equine (horse) estrogens for 25 days of the month. This dose of estrogen has been shown to be the lowest that prevents postmenopausal bone loss and is a much lower dose than that in oral contraceptives. The woman is examined after 1 to 2 months on this program and then at least every 6 months. Many women will have a return of their periods. Endometrial sampling may be repeated every year or two, although many gynecologists now omit endometrial sampling from the management of women who take progestins. Obviously, in the woman who has had a hysterectomy, sampling is omitted. Is it worth all this effort? Ask any woman who suffers from osteoporosis!

SUMMARY

Scientific evidence has proven that estrogen-replacement therapy prevents bone loss and protects against osteoporotic fractures. We don't know yet whether calcium supplements have the same effect, but many suspect that they don't. Estrogens may also protect against coronary artery disease but can increase the risk of endometrial cancer, hypertension, and gallbladder disease. If a woman takes progesterone along with estrogen (usually estrogen for the first 21 to 25 days of the month along with progesterone during the second and third weeks), she has no increased risk of cancer of the uterus; however, the long-term effects of taking progesterone are still unknown. Although no evidence links estrogen with breast cancer, women with abnormal breast biopsies should avoid estrogen-replacement therapy. In connection with this, all menopausal women should have a mammogram.

In the conservative approach to estrogen therapy, you and your doctor first determine whether you are at high risk for osteoporosis and are unlikely to develop side effects from estrogen. Your doctor makes this risk assessment by looking at your family history or by measuring your bone density. Current research may lead to better hormonal replacement therapy in the next few years. One recent advance is the development of a transdermal system for administering estrogens and progestin. This method should avoid some of the side effects associated with estrogens taken orally.

The three most important weapons in the fight against osteoporosis are good nutrition, hormonal replacement therapy, and physical exercise. The next chapter talks about the role of exercise in preventing and treating osteoporosis.

8 CHAPTER

Exercising for Skeletal Health

This chapter introduces the concept of physical fitness, which is essential for good health. Because the goals of exercise for prevention and those for treatment differ, and because mechanical stress may result in fractures once bone mass has become critically low, exercises that help prevent osteoporosis are considered separately from exercises recommended once osteoporosis has been diagnosed. The most important goal for the nonosteoporotic woman is to achieve high peak bone mass and prevent rapid bone loss following menopause. For the osteoporotic woman, the goals of exercise include pain relief, psychological benefits, and correction of altered posture.

Physical fitness involves the optimal functioning of all the body's systems, not only of the musculoskeletal system. Much attention has been paid to fitness of the cardiovascular, pulmonary, and musculoskeletal systems. In our increasingly sedentary society, it is becoming more and more difficult to become and remain fit. Even athletes frequently become sedentary in later life. You maintain fitness only by making a personal commitment to pursue a lifelong program of vigorous exercise for your entire body. Some accomplish this by participating in sports. Others may exercise at home or in a spa. Still others are successful only if they are part of a group exercise program that features social interaction as well as exercise. To gain an understanding of the physiological rudiments of conditioning, take a look at one of the many books on fitness, such as *Physiology of Fitness* (Sharkey, 1984).

The four components to fitness are muscular strength, muscular endurance, flexibility, and cardiorespiratory endurance. The first three are important for maintaining the musculoskeletal system in optimal condition. Muscle strength is the ability of a muscle to exert a force against resistance. This is measured by the amount of weight you can lift. Muscular endurance is the ability of a muscle to contract repeatedly (rowing on a rowing machine) or to hold a fixed contraction for a period of time (hanging from a parallel bar). Flexibility refers to your ability to move a muscle through its full range of motion. Flexibility prevents falling and also helps break a fall. Cardiorespiratory endurance is optimal functioning of the heart, lungs, and blood vessels both at rest and during exercise. This last component of exercise has received the most attention and is believed to be the most important for human survival. However, you can attain cardiorespiratory fitness without achieving the first three components of exercise. Similarly, you can develop and maintain muscular strength and endurance by lifting weights without improving your cardiorespiratory endurance.

AEROBIC AND STRENGTHENING EXERCISES

The major emphasis in recent years on fitness has been on attaining cardiovascular fitness in the hope of preventing death from heart attack. Thus, *aerobic exercise*, or aerobics, has been emphasized. Aerobic exercises use large-muscle groups in repetitious, rhythmic, nonstop movement for an extended period of time. In aerobic exercises the muscles use oxygen to carry out the exercise. Common aerobic exercises include walking, jogging, biking, swimming, and rowing.

There are three parts to any workout: the warm-up, the main conditioning period, and the cool-down. The warm-up prepares you for the vigorous part of the workout and stretches the muscles and tendons. The main conditioning period may consist of brisk walking, running, bicycling, skipping rope, or aerobic dancing. The cool-down involves tapering off the activity and is usually done by performing the main conditioning exercises at a lower intensity and then repeating the stretching exercises done in the warm-up.

The effectiveness of aerobic exercise can be monitored by heart rate. The heart rate range you will want to reach and maintain during your exercise period can be determined by a commonly used formula (Wilmoth, 1988). First, subtract your age (years) from 220 (222 represents the heart's anatomical and physiological limits). For a 60-year-old this part of the formula would look like this:

$$220 - 60 = 160$$

From the remainder, 160, you subtract the resting heart rate. Let's say in this case the resting heart rate is 80 beats per minute.

$$160 - 80 = 80$$

To stress the cardiovascular system, you should work out at between 65% and 85% of your maximum heart rate reserve. Use these values to determine the heart rate range:

$$80 \times .65 = 52 \text{ and } 80 \times .85 = 68$$

The individual's resting heart rate is added to this answer:

$$52 + 80 = 132 \text{ and } 68 + 80 = 148$$

The training range for an individual with these values would be between 132 and 148 beats per minute. Select the lower target rate.

Heart rate is measured by taking your pulse during the exercise. The pulse is best taken at the thumb side of the wrist with your middle and index fingers. Count the beats for 6 seconds and add a zero. Maintaining this target heart rate for 15 minutes three times per week will result in cardiorespiratory fitness. Aerobic exercise should be included in all fitness programs.

Strengthening Exercises

Calisthenic exercises and *isometric exercises* are types of anaerobic exercise, meaning "in the absence of oxygen." Calisthenics improve flexibility and strength and include such exercises as sit-ups and knee bends. They should be included in your exercise program and may be useful in your warm-ups and cool-downs. Isometrics and other anaerobic exercises are less useful and are generally not included in most fitness programs. Isometric exercises improve muscle strength and tone and involve placing tension on muscles with no movement. They do not improve cardiorespiratory fitness. An example of this type of exercise involves clasping your hands and pulling them apart without moving your hands or arms.

Anaerobic exercises are similar to aerobics but are done at a higher intensity for a shorter period of time. Anaerobic and isometric exercises may be dangerous for people with heart disease. Jogging several miles is aerobic, and the 50-meter dash is anaerobic.

FOUR COMPONENTS OF AN EFFECTIVE EXERCISE PROGRAM

There are four basic components of any physical fitness program: (a) intensity, (b) duration, (c) frequency, and (d) mode. Intensity refers to the level of exertion, whereas duration is the length of exertion. Frequency refers to the number of workouts per week and mode to the type of activity.

Below are the recommendations of the American College of Sports Medicine for the quantity and quality of training to maintain fitness:

- Frequency: 3 to 5 days per week
- Intensity: 60% to 90% of maximum heart rate reserve (determined by taking pulse during exercise)
- Duration: 15 to 60 minutes of continuous aerobic activity, depending on the intensity of the exercise
- Mode: Activity that uses large-muscle groups, that can be performed continuously, and that is rhythmic and aerobic

Whether you are developing your own fitness program, or thinking of joining a program at a health club, you should make sure these components are a part of the regimen.

EXERCISE RECOMMENDATIONS FOR SKELETAL HEALTH

It is doubtful that the aerobic exercises that produce cardiopulmonary fitness by being performed for 15 minutes three times per week place sufficient strain on the skeleton to prevent osteoporosis. At Brookhaven National Laboratory we (Aloia, Cohn, Ostuni, Cane, & Ellis, 1978b) studied a group of postmenopausal volunteers who exercised as a group for 1 hour, three times per week. Because these women were postmenopausal, we would have expected to see a decrease in bone mass. The exercises were recommended by the President's Council on Physical Fitness. There was an increase rather than the expected decrease in bone mass in these women after 1 year of exercise. The group was small, and the study was not carried out beyond a year; therefore, these results are preliminary.

Other researchers have studied or are currently studying similar types of exercise programs. One group is studying the benefits of class dancing. Another is studying exercise with Nautilus machines, which provide uniform resistance to the force that muscles exert throughout their ranges of motion. Preliminary reports from these studies suggest that the exercise programs are effective in preventing postmenopausal bone loss.

Until all these studies are completed, the kind of exercises we use in our program at the Winthrop Osteoporosis Center are recommended to be performed six to seven times per week. This program, if carried out in a home gym or a health spa, should be beneficial in preventing osteoporosis. (This program will be explained in the next section.) These exercises must be preceded and followed with calisthenics that stretch ligaments, increase flexibility, and improve balance. In addition, the pulse should be taken during the bicycling period of the program with a goal of reaching 70% of the maximal heart rate. In this way the exercise program will be beneficial to maintaining cardiorespiratory endurance as well as flexibility, muscular strength, and endurance.

Exercise Goals

It is important to appreciate that there are goals of an antifracture exercise program besides building bone mass. Exercise can improve posture. Having strong muscles can cushion a fall and prevent fracture. Increasing agility and balance can prevent falls. The confidence that develops in a fit individual is also protective against falling. The goals of a fracture-preventive, not an osteoporotic, exercise program follow:

- To attain maximal peak bone mass
- To prevent bone loss due to aging
- To maintain joint mobility
- To improve coordination
- To increase muscle mass
- To maintain posture
- To attain cardiorespiratory fitness
- To build confidence

Remember that exercise can be hazardous. The exercise we use for preventing osteoporosis may cause a fracture in a woman who already has osteoporosis. Older individuals (or those with any illness) should consult a physician before starting an exercise program. Moreover, if you are injured, you may become immobilized (the opposite of your goal) in a cast or be unable to exercise because of pain.

Exercise Precautions

Before beginning an exercise program, consult your physician, start slowly, and do not choose a hazardous program. Ideally, the exercise programs should be supervised by someone with expertise in physical medicine to minimize the risk of injury. Ten tips for any successful exercise program follow.

Ten Tips for a
Successful Exercise Program

1. See your physician before starting a formal program.
2. Start with brisk walking.
3. Exercise six to seven times per week for at least 30 minutes.
4. Unless you live in an ideal climate, exercise indoors.
5. Choose a program that you will enjoy. Join a spa or an exercise group; exercise to music.
6. Exercise in a comfortable, lightweight, loose-fitting outfit.
7. Take a tepid shower (not hot or cold) after exercising.
8. Whenever exercise is interrupted by illness or injury, resume your program at a lower level.
9. Increase your program slowly. Do not push beyond pleasant fatigue from which you can recover in a few minutes.
10. Keep a log of exercise. Include the date, type and time of exercise, and heart rate achieved.

Finally, a realistic appraisal of the relative value of exercise is important. Young women who run may develop amenorrhea (cessation of menstrual flow). These women have estrogen deficiency and actually develop reduced bone mass as an indirect result of high levels of physical activity. Obviously, if amenorrhea develops, premenopausal women should reduce their level of activity. However, there is another insight obtained from the low bone mass that develops from exercise-induced amenorrhea: Estrogen is a more potent factor than is exercise in regulating bone mass in women.

If we were to weigh the relative importance of each factor in postmenopausal bone loss, estrogen would influence bone loss three times as much as exercise would under ordinary conditions. Thus, although exercise is important in developing and maintaining a healthy skeleton, the dictum "Nothing in excess" must be remembered. Another way of viewing low bone mass from estrogen deficiency resulting from exercise is that there are interactions between the various factors that affect bone mass. If strenuous exercise is initiated, adjustments should be made in caloric intake. It has also been recently observed that the beneficial effects of exercise are achieved only if dietary calcium intake is adequate. Diet, estrogens, and exercise should be considered a team in the fight against osteoporosis.

A HOME GYM PREVENTIVE EXERCISE PROGRAM

This program, developed at Winthrop University Hospital with Brookhaven National Laboratory, emphasizes resistance rather than free-limb exercises such as calisthenics or yoga. Resistance exercises are based on the belief that the mechanical load placed on bone is the factor that results in increased bone mass.

One training device is a stationary bicycle with adjustable pedal resistance. Assume you have had little physical training in the past and wish to begin at a safe level. Set the pedal resistance to the lowest level and time yourself for 1 minute of pedaling at a moderate pace. Each day, increase the time 5 seconds until you can pedal for 5 minutes continuously. Then increase the pedal resistance one notch and start with 2 minutes. Once again, add 5 seconds per day until you can pedal for 5 minutes, working up to 15 minutes in the manner just described. Stop if you experience pain or when you feel you have reached a level of fatigue and effort from which it will take 2 to 3 minutes to recover.

Another recommended training device is the rowing machine. Here again, the degree of resistance is adjustable. Start with the lowest tension and perform 10 rows. Add 1 repetition each week until you can perform 25 rows. Then increase the resistance one notch and start over with 10 repetitions, working up to 25 in the same manner.

With the home equipment described above, you could, in time, put sufficient positive stress on the musculoskeletal system to minimize bone loss. The important point is to be consistent. The exercises should be performed at least six times per week, and daily exercise is preferred. Follow this routine at the same time each day you exercise. These exercises should be preceded by calisthenics and postural and positional exercises and should *not* be done by women who have osteoporosis as the exercises are for prevention only. A detailed exercise program follows.

The Preventive Home Program

This is an outline of the program I often recommend to my patients for their use at home.

Warm-Up

Warming up should begin no more than 15 minutes before the workout. Gentle stretching and calisthenic-type exercises should be performed for at least 3 to 5 minutes. Each major muscle group should be stretched before working out. All the exercises in this section of the program are standing exercises.

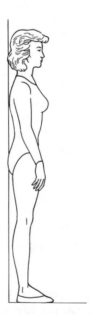

Stand tall.   Stand with your back against a wall; squeeze your shoulder blades together, tighten your abdominal muscles, try to place your lower back against the wall, and lift your head high. *Repeat 10 times.*

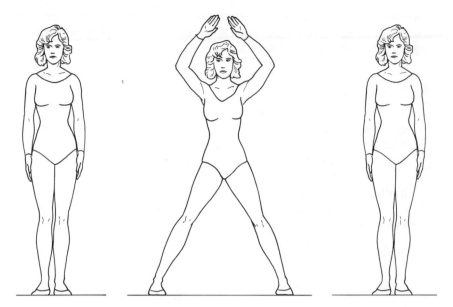

Jumping Jacks.   Swing your arms over your head and spread your feet apart in one movement. Then return to the starting position. *Repeat 20 times.*

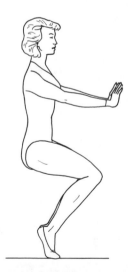

Knee bends.   Keep your back erect and bend your knees into a partial squatting position. Then return to the starting position. *Repeat 10 times.*

The core of the program is the workout. Never begin the workout until the warm-up has been completed. If you do a proper warm-up, your risk for injury is small.

Workout

The workout is intended to strengthen and condition. These exercises are done on the floor and with a stationary bicycle and rowing machine. Please note that for aerobic conditioning you must exercise for at least fifteen minutes in your target heart range. Exercising for a longer duration will place more load on your skeletal system. However, duration, like intensity, should be increased gradually. The suggested times and number of repetitions here are only suggestions. If you become very fatigued, breathless, or dizzy, stop.

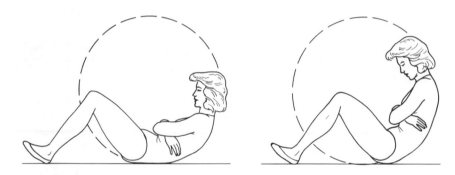

Sit-ups.   Lie on your back with the knees bent and hands across your stomach. Raise your head and trunk to an upright position and hold for 1 count. *Repeat 20 times.*

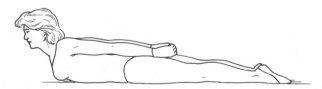

Back extensions.   Lie on the floor with your face down; extend your body from above the waist. *Repeat 15 times.*

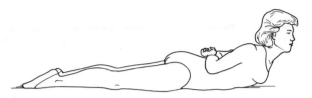

Back tighteners.   Lie on the floor with your face down and hands folded over the lower-back area. Raise your head and chest and tense the *gluteus maximus* and the lower-back muscles (do not hyperextend). *Repeat 15 times.*

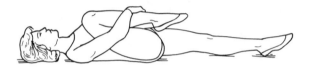

Lower back stretch.   Lie on your back, lift and bend one leg, and pull down the knee to the chest. Repeat with the other leg. *Repeat 10 times.*

Bicycling.   *5 minutes.*

Rowing machine.   *25 rows.*

The last section of the program, cooling down, is just as important as warming up in avoiding injury.

Cool-Down

During the cool-down your heart rate will return gradually to its usual rate. You can again stretch your muscles to avoid cramping. The cool-down should last at least 3 to 5 minutes. In cooling down, speed is not the objective.

Knee bends.   Keep your back erect and bend your knees into a partial squatting position. Then return to the starting position. *Repeat 10 times* (see page 139).

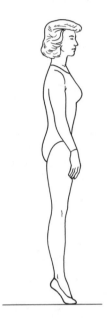

Heel raises.   With your feet apart, raise to a toe position, then lower your body. *Repeat 15 times.*

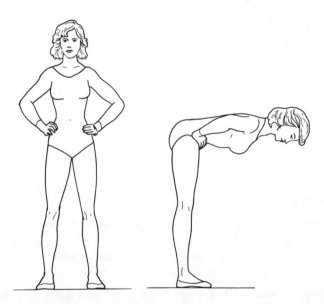

Forward bend.   Stand astride with your hands on your hips and bend slowly to a 90-degree angle. Return slowly to an erect position. *Repeat 10 times.*

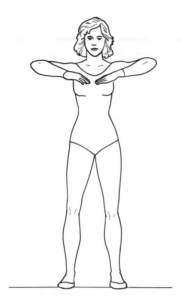

Shoulder-and-chest stretch.   Stand astride with your arms at shoulder level and elbows bent. Force the elbows backward and return to the starting position. *Repeat 10 times.*

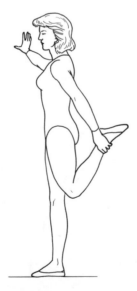

Front leg stretch.   Stand erect and pull the ankle of one leg to the hip and hold for 20 seconds. Repeat using the other side. *Repeat 2 times.*

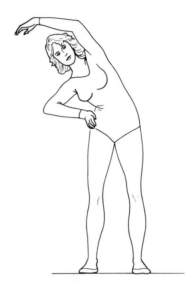

Side stretch.   Bend your trunk to the right with the left arm stretched overhead, then use the same procedure for the other side. *Repeat 10 times.*

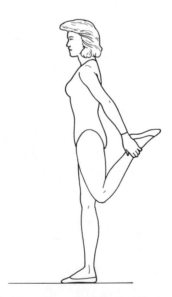

Position control—A.   Stand with the fingers supporting first one leg and then the other. *Repeat on each leg for 10 counts, then repeat on each leg for 20 counts.*

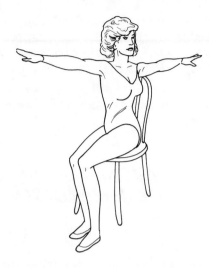

Position control—B. Sitting on a chair, turn and look to the left and to the right. Repeat with your arms stretched sideways. *Perform each 10 times.*

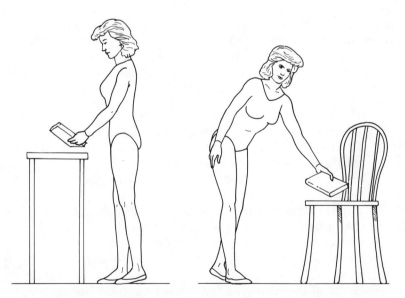

Position control—C. Stand and slowly pick up an object from a table. Place it on a chair and then back on the table. *Repeat each 10 times.*

Stand tall.   Stand with your back against the wall. Squeeze your shoulder blades together, tighten your abdominal muscles, try to place your lower back against the wall, and lift your head high. *Repeat 10 times* (see page 138).

Remember regular exercise will provide you with many benefits—skeletal and cardiovascular health and a renewed sense of confidence in your body.

PHYSICAL TRAINING FOR THE ELDERLY

The risks of an exercise program are obviously greater in the elderly. The major concerns are *cardiac arrhythmia* (an abnormal heart rhythm) or musculoskeletal injuries. Indeed, some group programs for senior citizens have reported as high as a 50% rate of musculoskeletal injuries during the first few weeks of exercise. One of the consequences of such an early injury is to discourage both the injured individual and his or her group from continuing with the program.

There are many factors that may contribute to this high injury rate. As discussed in chapter 4, elderly individuals have a decreased sense of balance and may have muscle weakness. The tendons become shortened after many years of inactivity. There is an impaired ability to break a fall. The following factors may lead to injury in a training program in any age group and are also frequently found when an older individual is injured:

- Obesity may be present.
- The warm-up period may be inadequate.
- The calisthenics may be too vigorous, with twisting movements and too much stretching.
- Progression from one step to the next in a program may be too rapid.
- The exercise period may be continued beyond the phase when the individual feels pleasantly fatigued.
- Exercise may be on a hard or dangerous surface.
- Shoes with inadequate heels and poor ankle support may be used.
- Physical impairments may make exercise hazardous.

Before beginning an exercise program, the elderly should consult their physicians and may undergo an exercise stress test to determine whether they have coronary artery disease. If the test is positive, then exercise may initially be performed with cardiac monitoring. A hypertensive response to a stress test (the blood pressure rises with exercise) requires an adjustment in antihypertensive medication.

It is important not to neglect the value of increasing fitness through the activities of daily living. Walking the dog, mowing the lawn, and climbing the stairs are all good forms of exercise. In an exercise program, you can monitor these activities by keeping an activity diary.

EXERCISE RECOMMENDATIONS FOR OSTEOPOROTIC WOMEN

One of the first steps in an exercise program for someone who has suffered a fracture is to overcome an abnormal fear of fracture. Some women are confined to their homes not because of pain but because of fear. On the other hand, prudence is important as undue stress on the spine must be avoided, or a spinal fracture may occur. The goals of an exercise program for women with osteoporosis follow:

- To restore confidence
- To maintain joint mobility
- To improve coordination
- To improve posture
- To reduce pain
- To increase muscle strength
- To prevent bone loss
- To attain cardiorespiratory fitness

Never do exercises that flex your spine (bending forward at the waist). In one study (Sinaki & Mikkelsen, 1984), it was found that spinal flexion exercises cause fractures in osteoporotic women. Eighteen of 28 women developed aggravations of their vertebral fractures when they were in a program using spinal flexion exercises as compared to only 4 of 25 when these exercises were avoided.

A HOME OSTEOPOROSIS EXERCISE PROGRAM

As initial exercise, I recommend walking for 5 minutes in an area with even surfaces. One minute per week is added until you are walking 20 minutes without stopping. This can be done twice a day. Your eventual goal may be walking 3 miles per day. I also recommend swimming initially because it does not strain the skeleton yet improves joint mobility and restores confidence. It is likely that weight-bearing exercises (including walking) are preferable for preventing bone loss, but a recent study suggests that swimming may also increase bone mass.

Following this initial period, specific exercises are recommended. Remember to avoid exercises that flex the spine. The types of exercise that are useful are

- back extension,
- pectoral stretching,
- deep breathing,
- abdominal muscle strengthening,
- exercises that increase the strength in the *lumbar extensor muscles* and the gluteus maximus, and
- exercises that improve posture and coordination.

Although you must remember to avoid injury to your skeleton, these exercises will often both reduce pain and produce a feeling of well-being. It is amazing to observe the atrophy in the muscles and ligaments of osteoporotic women caused by disuse. Check with your physician before you begin an exercise program, and begin gradually. Also, pay continuous attention to your posture and avoid stooping. I recommend, in addition to walking, that women with osteoporosis gradually perform the exercises in this chapter every morning and evening. Start slowly and increase the level of activity each week by 10% to 15%. You may begin an exercise that requires 20 counts with only 1 or 2 counts.

The Home Program for Osteoporotic Women

This is an outline of the program I often recommend to my osteoporotic patients for home use. I do not divide this program into warm-up, workout, and cool-down sections because I encourage women with osteoporosis to always exercise gradually. Exercising quickly in the case of an osteoporotic woman is not an affirmation of health; rather it is an invitation to injury.

Standing Exercises

These exercises increase strength, flexibility, and position control.

Stand tall.   Stand with your back against the wall; squeeze your shoulder blades together, tighten your abdominal muscles, try to place your lower back against the wall, and lift your head high. *Repeat 10 times* (see page 138).

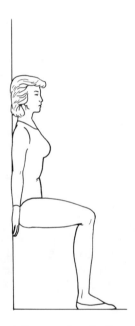

Wall slide.   Stand with your back flat against the wall and your heels away from the wall. Pull your chin in. Slide down the wall several inches and then straighten up. At a safe pace, increase the depth to which you bend. It may help to keep a rolled towel in the small of your back. *Repeat 20 times.*

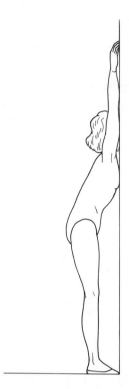

Wall arch.   Turn around and face the wall with your arms stretched upward as high as possible and your arms and toes touching the wall. Arch your back away from the wall in a comfortable position while keeping your arms and chest against the wall; stretch your arms as high as they will go, then move your feet away from the wall. *Repeat 20 times.*

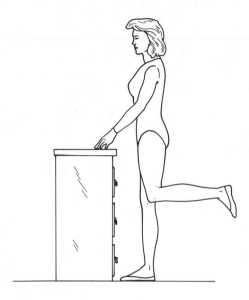

Position control—A.   Stand with a hand resting on a tabletop or a low chest of drawers. Stand on one leg and then the other. *Repeat on each leg for 10 counts.*

Position control—B.   Sitting on a chair, turn and look to the left and the right. Repeat with your arms stretched sideways. Repeat with your hands behind the head and with the elbows pointing out. *Perform each 10 times* (see page 145).

Position control—C.   Stand and slowly pick up an object from a table. Place it on a chair and then back on the table. *Repeat each 10 times* (see page 145).

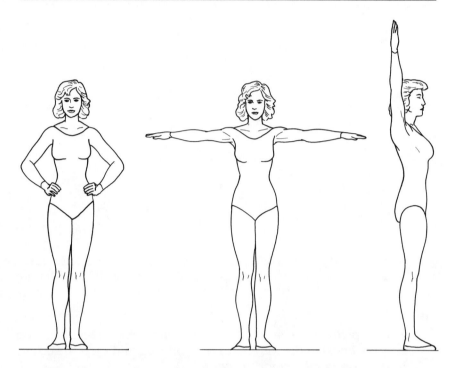

Back extension pectoral stretching.   In succession (a) place your hands on hips, (b) raise your arms parallel to floor with the palms down and stretch shoulders backward, (c) reach up over your head (arms perpendicular to floor), (d) return your hands to hips, and inhale as deeply as possible and then exhale slowly. *Repeat 20 times.* This exercise can be performed sitting in a chair.

Stationary bicycle.   Ride a stationary bicycle for 15 minutes. Rest your hands on the seat (do not lean forward). Build up to this level in the way described for the exercises that help prevent osteoporosis and attain your target heart rate. If the seat of the bicycle is uncomfortable, use a foam-rubber cushion.

Bed Exercises

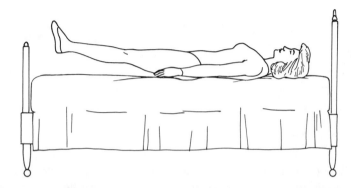

Abdominal strengthening exercise.   Raise your legs off the bed 10 degrees with the knees extended (straight). *Repeat 20 times.*

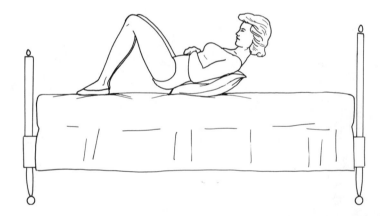

Head up.   With your knees flexed, raise your head. It may first be necessary to push up with your arms. Later, your hands should remain on the abdomen. You may need to place a pillow under the small of your back. *Repeat 20 times.* This exercise partially flexes the spine. If it causes discomfort, consult your physician.

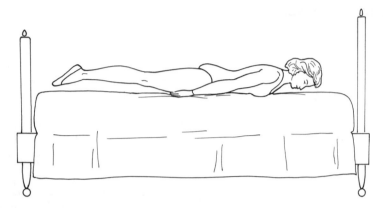

Gentle prone lift.   Lie flat with your hands under your thighs. Raise your head, shoulders, and legs from bed, then return to the starting position. *Repeat 20 times.*

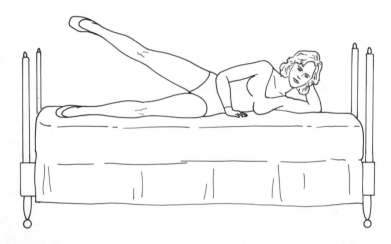

Leg raise.   With the left side of your body on the bed and your head resting on the left arm, lift your right leg 12 to 24 inches off the bed, then lower it. Use your right hand to support your body. Repeat on the right side. *Repeat 20 (10 for each leg) times.*

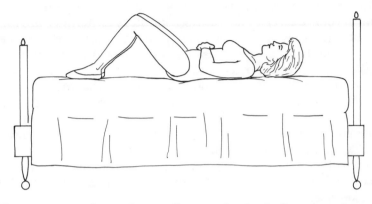

Gluteus exercise. Lying flat on the bed, flex your knees. Press the small of your back against the bed by tensing your buttocks and stomach muscles. Hold tight for 5 seconds. *Repeat 20 times.*

Stand tall. *Repeat the first stand-tall exercise 10 times.* Now walk forward and try to maintain this posture. You may repeat walking with a pillow on your head several times a day to practice good posture.

Most women can perform this exercise program. Some women may need to place a pillow behind their heads and under the smalls of their backs when they start. Women who wear braces or corsets may have to wear these devices when they begin the exercise program. I usually recommend increasing the amount of exercise on a weekly basis until the above program is achieved. The speed at which an exercise is completed is unimportant for our purposes. Thus, in the first week, each of the above exercises are performed only twice, once in the morning and once in the evening. The stationary bicycle is used with no resistance for 2 minutes in the morning and 2 minutes in the evening. During the second week, each exercise is performed twice in the morning and twice in the evening and is increased gradually until the full program is achieved.

SUMMARY

Physical fitness is essential for good health. Having a fit musculoskeletal system can prevent osteoporotic fractures by attaining peak bone mass, reducing postmenopausal bone loss, and preventing injuries. The four components of fitness are muscular strength, muscular endurance, flexibility, and cardiorespiratory endurance.

The first three are important for preventing osteoporotic fractures, and aerobic exercises for cardiorespiratory endurance are included in all fitness programs because of their importance in preventing death from heart attack. This chapter reviewed an exercise program designed to prevent osteoporotic fractures, while at the same time cautioning elderly women about the injuries that might result from an exercise program. Younger women who exercise to the extreme of developing menstrual irregularities (exercise-induced amenorrhea) may actually have a greater risk of osteoporosis because they are deficient in estrogens. If exercise results in estrogen deficiency, there will be a decrease in peak bone mass. Finally, if you don't take in an adequate amount of calcium, you won't realize the full benefits of exercise.

If you already have osteoporosis, you should exercise for reasons other than its effect on bone mass: to restore confidence, maintain joint mobility, improve coordination, improve posture, reduce pain, and attain cardiorespiratory fitness. You can attain all of these goals without the risk of injury. However, the type of exercise that stimulates bone formation to such a degree that it increases bone mass is hazardous. If your bone mass is low, strenuous weight-bearing exercises may result in fractures. It is important for you to understand the difference between the two programs of exercise. A weight-lifting workout is not beneficial if you have osteoporosis. Always avoid flexing the spine. An ideal form of exercise for osteoporotic women is walking, which attains all four components of fitness.

Chapters 6 through 8 discussed the three weapons you can use to combat osteoporosis: diet, estrogen, and exercise. The next chapter considers tests used in evaluating osteoporosis and discusses treatment strategies for individuals with osteoporosis.

9 CHAPTER

Diagnostic Testing

Whether you already have osteoporosis or are simply approaching menopause, your doctor may request a number of tests to determine your skeletal health. This chapter discusses the techniques that health care professionals currently use to measure bone mass. These techniques are used to choose women for estrogen-replacement therapy and evaluate the effectiveness of drug treatment for osteoporosis. The chapter also discusses other tests that are used in the treatment of menopausal women and in the evaluation of the causes of osteoporosis.

BONE MASS MEASUREMENT

Since the development of methods that have enabled us to accurately measure bone mass, a virtual explosion of knowledge about osteoporosis has occurred. It's not possible to simply look at an X ray of the spine and determine whether the bone is normal or osteoporotic. A *radiologist* would not be sure that you had spinal osteoporosis unless he or she observed deformity of the vertebra indicating that a fracture had occurred. The woman with a vertebral fracture has at least 20% to 30% less bone mass than the average young adult. Fortunately, new quantitative methods can detect low bone mass at an earlier stage, and repeated measurements can be made to determine the rate of bone gain or loss.

Although some researchers would argue that I am ignoring the new techniques, this chapter deals with only those methods that are currently available. These include *radiographic morphometry*; total body *neutron activation analysis* with whole-body counting; *photon absorptiometry*, including single-photon absorptiometry of the radius and dual-photon absorptiometry and *quantitative digital radiography* of the spine and femur; and computerized axial tomography (CAT), more accurately called *computed tomography*, of the spine. These tests are painless, safe, and don't involve injection of dyes or radioactive substances.

RADIOGRAPHIC MORPHOMETRY

Although radiographic morphometry is the least suitable technique available, it uses X rays and is available wherever there is an X-ray machine. The most frequently used measurement is of the multiple bones of the hand, or the *metacarpals*. The widths of the second, third, and fourth metacarpal bones are measured in both hands and then averaged. The difficulty in putting the hand in the same position each time makes repeat measurements imprecise. Moreover, the bones measured are composed primarily of cortical bone. There is a poor correlation between the metacarpal index and bone volume of the spine.

TOTAL BODY NEUTRON ACTIVATION ANALYSIS AND WHOLE-BODY COUNTING

This is the only available technique that measures the amount of calcium in the skeleton (98% of the body's calcium is in the skeleton). Unfortunately, this technique requires elaborate and expensive equipment to expose patients to only low levels of radiation and to be precise. It is available only in a few centers in the world, with the most advanced facility developed at Brookhaven National Laboratory. It is considered the "gold standard" in bone-mineral measurement.

Patients are exposed to *neutrons* (a form of radiation that is different from X rays) that interact with the calcium in the body. For a few minutes, the body's calcium emits radiation that is measured in a whole-body counter (counts are units of radioactivity). The same procedure is carried out with a *phantom* (a model that contains a known amount of calcium). The radiation emitted by the patient is compared to that emitted by the phantom. It is thus possible to determine the exact amount of calcium in a patient's body (e.g., 628 grams). Measurements may then be repeated every 6 months to determine whether the patient is gaining or losing bone.

SINGLE-PHOTON ABSORPTIOMETRY

In this method a radioactive material emits another type of radiation: photons. The amount of radiation that passes through the bone being measured (usually the radius) is proportional to the amount of bone mineral in its path. The forearm is placed flat on the instrument with the radiation source beneath the forearm. A counter (or scanner) on the other side of the forearm moves over (scans) the bone so that the radiation transmitted is compared to a phantom of known bone-mineral content per centimeter scanned. Other bones may be measured, including the ulna and the finger, but the radius is used most frequently.

Measurements are more accurate when little muscle and fat tissue surround the bone. Different sites on the radius may be measured. There is more trabecular bone near the distal (wrist) end of the radius. Some investigators believe that the more distal sites may more accurately reflect the trabecular bone mineral content of the spine. This has led to measurement of an "ultradistal" site. Any of these sites may be used, and measurements usually take less than 20 minutes. Most experts, though, prefer to measure bone density in the sites most likely to fracture—the spine and the hip.

DUAL-PHOTON ABSORPTIOMETRY

In this method a radioactive material is used that emits photons at two different energies. The principle is the same as that for single-photon absorptiometry, but using the two energies allows one to subtract the soft-tissue (nonskeletal) component. The most frequently measured area is L2 through L4 (i.e., lumbar vertebrae L2, L3, and L4).

More recently, dual-photon absorptiometry has been used to measure the density of the femur (hip) and may also scan the entire skeleton to assess total body bone-mineral content. This technique has been used in many research centers and is now available commercially. A thousand units were in use in the United States in 1989. The procedure is similar to single-photon absorptiometry. The patient simply lies on a table while the scanning piece passes over the area of interest (femur or spine) or the whole body. Representative scans of the whole body, spine, and femur are depicted in Figures 9.1, 9.2, and 9.3. One of the difficulties with measuring bone density of the spine with dual photon absorptiometry is that the technique measures all the calcium in its path. For example, if there are bone changes from arthritis or there is calcification in the aorta (a blood vessel that is in front of the spine), that calcium will be included in the measurement.

An advance in dual-photon absorptiometry called quantitative digital radiography was introduced in late 1987. This technique uses an X-ray tube instead of radioactive material and has better reproducibility and a slightly lower radioactive exposure. The amount of time necessary to complete a scan is also less.

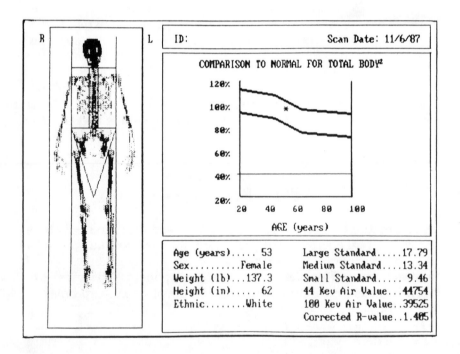

Figure 9.1 A whole body scan with the computer report that displays the patient's value on a graph for comparison with normal values.

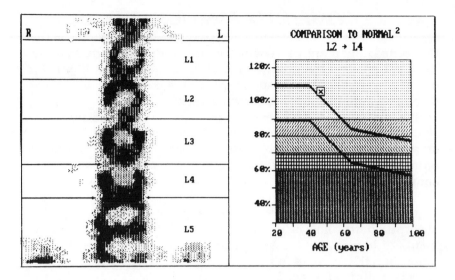

Figure 9.2 A spine scan with a computer generated graph comparing the patient's value to individuals of the same race and age.

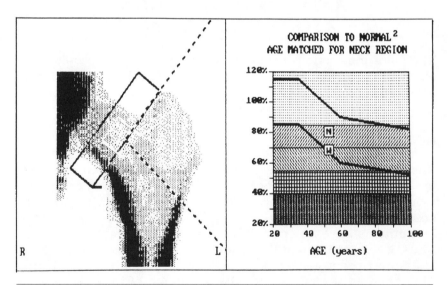

Figure 9.3 A scan of the neck of the femur. Two areas are given in the graph. The neck and femur (N) and Ward's Triangle (W). This latter area may be important in the development of hip fracture.

COMPUTED TOMOGRAPHY

Computed tomography has revolutionized radiology in recent years. The CAT scan is available in most of the larger community hospitals. It is applied to the measurement of the spine's bone mass, again through comparison with a known standard. The major advantage of this method is that trabecular bone can be analyzed separately from cortical bone. However, the CAT scan may not be measuring only bone mineral and may be less accurate than the other techniques. The various techniques for measuring bone mineral are compared in Table 9.1.

The CAT scan is less accurate in older people. Furthermore, it requires a much higher radiation exposure than does photon absorptiometry. This is important to consider if repeated measurements of bone-mineral levels are planned. Nonetheless, in 1988 more than 800 centers in the United States were measuring bone density with CAT scans.

ANSWERS TO QUESTIONS ABOUT DENSITOMETRY

The following sections will address questions many people have about the accuracy, safety, and comparative risks and benefits of each type of densitometry test.

Reproducibility

The methods of *bone densitometry* described so far can be used for the diagnosis of low bone mass but are also important for monitoring changes in bone mass (with or without treatment). Suppose that 1% of bone mass is lost in 1 year. The most sophisticated instruments have an error of measurement of greater than 1%. Thus, if a measurement is repeated the next day, changes of 2% to 3% may occur just from the technical error of the instrument. This amount of error due to the technique of measurement is referred to as the reproducibility of a measurement.

One way to minimize the effects of measurement errors is to perform frequent measurements of bone mineral. If measurements were made every week, it would take only a few months to determine whether bone density was increasing or decreasing. This frequency of measurements, however, is impractical because of cost,

Table 9.1 Comparison of Techniques to Measure Bone Mineral

Method	Accuracy	Reproducibility error	Radiation exposure (mrad)	Predominant bone type
Radiogrammetry	10%	5%	<100	Cortical
Computed tomography	<10%	3%	250	Cortical and trabecular separately
Photon absorptiometry				
Single	1%	2%	5	Cortical
Dual (radioisotope source)	5%	2%	10	Trabecular
Dual (quantitative digital radiography)		1%	<3	Trabecular
Neutron activation analysis	1%	2%	28	Total

radiation dose, and inconvenience. A reasonable compromise is to repeat the measurement every 6 months. Generally, after five bi-annual measurements (2 years) with photon absorptiometry, it can safely be said that any changes observed are actual changes in bone mass rather than those due to measurement error.

Repeated bone measurements may be taken to identify women who are rapid losers of bone mass. If estrogen is not recommended at the time of menopause, an excessively rapid rate of bone loss can be detected over the next 1½ years. Estrogen replacement can then be recommended to the 20% to 30% of women who have an ade-quate peak bone mass but develop osteoporosis as a result of more rapid than usual postmenopausal bone loss. Unfortunately, repeat measurements are impractical in terms of their cost.

Is Radiation Exposure Safe?

As a result of much publicity in the media, many individuals are concerned about unnecessary radiation exposure. Obviously, unnecessary radiation should be avoided. However, the decisions we make in life involve two factors: possible risk and possible benefit. Physicians refer to this as the risk-to-benefit ratio of diag-nostic techniques and of treatment modalities. If you have acute appendicitis, there is a risk from anesthesia if you have surgery. However, the benefits of an operation (which is lifesaving) far out-weigh the risks involved. The risk from radiation exposure from the methods described is so small compared to the potential benefit that there should be no hesitation to make bone-mineral measurements. The radiation dose from a dual photon measurement of the spine is similar to that received from background radiation flying an air-plane from New York to Denver! (See Table 9.1 for radiation doses.)

Which Technique Is Preferable?

The choice of technique for bone-mineral measurements often de-pends on what is available within the community in which the patient resides. Measurement of total body bone-mineral density with dual-photon absorptiometry provides similar information to total body calcium, but the procedure currently takes a long time (45 minutes) to perform. A CAT scan of the spine has the dis-advantage of higher radiation exposures. There is little evidence that measurement at a site closer to the wrist improves single-photon absorptiometry measurements. Moreover, there is a growing consensus that, if one is interested in spinal osteoporosis, the vertebrae should be measured, and if one is interested in the risk of hip fracture, the hip should be measured. Dual-photon absorptiometry of the spine and hip show that bone loss from these skeletal sites begins before menopause, and this may be the reason why this measurement will be more useful in detecting women at risk than will measurement at the radius (wrist).

Sometimes a single measurement of the radius or spine may be misleading. For example, the radius of a tennis player may not reflect the mass of the total skeleton because of a local increase in bone volume from repeated strain on the forearm. Conversely, a paralyzed upper extremity or one that has been immobilized for treatment of a fracture will have immobilization (disuse) osteoporosis, which may not be present in other parts of the skeleton. In addition, a variety of hormonal disorders may result in divergent changes in cortical and trabecular bone. This discordant response of cortical and trabecular bone to hormones may also occur following treatment of osteoporosis. Thus, in certain experimental forms of therapy, trabecular bone mass increased while cortical bone mass decreased. This has certainly been the case with fluoride treatment, where bone mineral may increase dramatically in the spine but decrease in the hip.

Therefore, in following up on the response to therapy, it is desirable to measure both cortical and trabecular bone mass and to measure changes in the whole skeleton or the particular regions of interest. This can be done by measuring both total body calcium (or total body bone mineral) and another site that measures either predominantly cortical or trabecular bone mass (dual-photon absorptiometry or CAT scan of the spine for trabecular bone and single-photon absorptiometry of the radius for cortical bone). It can also be done by measuring the density of the radius and the spine. It is my practice to measure the bone mineral of the radius and that of the lumbar spine and hip using both single- and dual-photon absorptiometry. For the research projects conducted by the Winthrop researchers at Brookhaven National Laboratory, neutron activation analysis is used as well and provides a comprehensive view of skeletal changes (including the total skeleton, radius, and spine). Measurements are made every 4 to 6 months for 2 years before an objective response to treatment in an individual can be evaluated.

What About the Expense?

Although some forms of bone densitometry have been in use for more than 2 decades for research purposes, only in the 1980s has an effort been made to make these instruments available to the general public. Thus, for the purpose of health insurance carriers, these measurements are considered "new technology." As a result of technological advances in medicine, health care costs have risen to the extent that government, unions, and business corporations (who pay health insurance companies for their employees) are unwilling to pay for tests unless they are found to be cost-effective (i.e., the increased costs can be justified by increased benefits). Unfortunately, public health care policy is influenced by many factors other than the value of a new technique. There is no question about the accuracy of bone densitometry; however, there is a question about who should pay for it.

The value of densitometry has been incorrectly questioned in the media as a result of the scientific community's reaction to commercial development of "storefront" densitometry centers. One such enterprise developed single-photon absorptiometry centers throughout the country in osteoporosis diagnostic clinics that had franchise agreements with local physicians. Such commercial ventures have been opposed or resented by some researchers and discussed in an exposé fashion on television news programs such as 20/20.

Densitometry is useful in assessing risk for osteoporosis at menopause and for monitoring the effects of drug treatment in women who already have osteoporosis. Mass screening is so costly that most health insurance carriers will probably never reimburse women who have this test. I believe that women who are at high risk by virtue of their medical histories should be reimbursed, but this too may not happen.

One use of bone densitometry is to detect at menopause the women who are at risk for the development of osteoporosis. This is done by comparing the individual's peak bone mass value with the average value for women aged 20 to 40. In this way the percentage reduction in bone density is calculated:

$$\text{Percent of normal} = \frac{\text{individual's value} \times 100}{\text{average value of peak bone mass}}$$

For example, a value of 76% of young normals indicates a reduction of 24% in bone density, which means that the individual is at high risk for fracture. The use of densitometry in this fashion is similar to using blood pressure to assess risk for heart attack or for stroke. High blood pressure suggests that efforts should be made to treat blood pressure levels. Low bone density means that intensive efforts must be made to prevent bone loss (or, ideally, to increase bone mass).

Who Should Undergo Bone Densitometry?

Some researchers believe that bone densitometry should not be used to assess the skeletal status and risk for osteoporosis in post-menopausal women. They correctly state that bone densitometry is imperfect in diagnosing osteoporosis and that there are factors in addition to bone density that make bone susceptible to fracture. These researchers have confused diagnosis with the assessment of skeletal status to estimate risk. Bone densitometry is a poor tool with which to discriminate among older women who do or do not have osteoporotic fractures because, currently, most older women have low bone mass. The main difference between a 90-year-old with and one without a hip fracture is whether or not they fell. On the other hand, those women with lower bone-density values at menopause are more likely to be at risk for future fracture.

Screening Perspectives

The concept of abnormal versus normal diseases should not be used with bone-density measurements. An example of an abnormal-normal disease is cancer. A biopsy may be used to determine that you either do or do not have cancer. The relationship between osteoporosis and fracture is more analagous to the relationship between high blood pressure and stroke. Some stroke victims have high blood pressure and others do not; you cannot diagnose stroke from a blood pressure measurement just as you cannot diagnose the presence of osteoporotic fractures from a bone-density measurement. However, the higher your blood pressure, the more likely you are to have a stroke in the future. Similarly, the lower your bone density, the more likely you are to suffer an osteoporotic fracture in the future. The reasonable approach to the use of bone densitometry lies midway between the extreme positions either that all Caucasian women should have bone-mineral measurement at menopause or that no women should undergo densitometry.

Mass Versus Selective Screening

The procedure of measuring bone density to select women for hormonal replacement therapy at menopause is referred to as *screening*. Mass screening refers to testing the entire population at risk (e.g., white women at menopause). Selective screening refers to performing densitometry to confirm low bone mass in only those individuals who are considered high risk by historical factors (e.g., the white, slender woman whose mother had osteoporosis, who smokes, is inactive, drinks moderately, never drank milk, had an early menopause, and takes steroid medication). Presently, mass screening is too costly, and selective screening should be performed only to help decide whether to begin estrogen-replacement therapy.

Presenting Screening Options

For those women who have already decided to either take or not take estrogens, densitometry is not needed as the outcome will not be altered. Similarly, knowledge of bone density does not influence the possible interventions for those women for whom the physician will not prescribe estrogen because of contraindications. However, women with an average or low risk for osteoporosis from historical factors may be given the option of densitometry of the spine (or perhaps the hip) to help them decide whether to take estrogen. Low bone density of the spine indicates a risk for osteoporosis in the next decade or so of life.

Most of the information provided thus far about osteoporosis refers to healthy women. It is important to remember that individuals with certain medical problems should have an assessment of skeletal status using densitometry. For example, prolonged bed rest causes osteoporosis, as does an overactive thyroid or taking certain medications. Patients in these high-risk categories may benefit from bone-mineral measurement.

Another time to measure bone density is when monitoring therapy in the older woman who already suffers from osteoporosis. If the patient or the physician has decided in advance that medication to treat osteoporosis will not be used, then there is no value in performing densitometry. On the other hand, measurement of bone mineral is the only way to tell whether medication is working. For those physicians and patients who are committed to aggressive therapy using medication, bone-mineral measurement is essential.

OTHER TESTS USED IN EVALUATING AND TREATING OSTEOPOROSIS

There are tests that are often performed on patients with osteoporosis that do not help diagnose primary osteoporosis but rather exclude other conditions that may have similar X-ray images. Common laboratory tests used in the diagnosis of osteoporosis are given in Table 9.2.

Each of these tests will be explained in the following sections.

Table 9.2   Laboratory Tests in Osteoporosis

Test	Detects
CBC	Anemia, high white blood count
Urinalysis	Proteinuria
Chem-screen	Liver or kidney disease Hyperparathyroidism Paget's disease Osteomalacia
Protein electrophoresis	Multiple myeloma
Serum thyroxine	Overactive thyroid

Note: Optional osteoporosis laboratory tests include a 24-hour urine-calcium to detect hypercalciuria, a 24-hour urine-hydroxyproline to detect high bone remodeling, and a serum osteocalcin, also to detect high bone remodeling.

Complete Blood Count (CBC)

The CBC is a blood test that helps diagnose anemia or abnormality of the white blood cells. Primary osteoporosis is associated with a normal CBC. An abnormal CBC may indicate secondary osteoporosis and more serious disorders such as *multiple myeloma*, a cancer of certain cells in the bone marrow.

Chem-Screen

This test is an automated chemical analysis that is performed on a single blood sample. As many as 24 different tests may be performed. The blood calcium is high in hyperparathyroidism and may be low in osteomalacia; it is normal in primary osteoporosis. This blood test will detect abnormalities in liver and kidney function that could produce osteoporosis. The *alkaline phosphatase* level is elevated in osteomalacia and hyperparathyroidism but is usually normal in osteoporosis (it may be elevated after a fracture).

Other Blood Tests

Because an overactive thyroid may cause osteoporosis, the level of thyroid hormone is usually tested. A *protein electrophoresis* is used to identify patients with multiple myeloma. Vitamin D levels may be measured to determine if supplementation is needed or if levels are so low that osteomalacia should be suspected. Parathyroid hormone levels may also be measured to look for evidence of hyperparathyroidism, malabsorption, or liver or kidney disease. Osteocalcin levels may be used to help identify women who have more rapid bone loss.

Urine Tests

A routine urinalysis is performed to look for *proteinuria* (an excess of protein in the urine), which may result from kidney disease or multiple myeloma. A 24-hour urine collection may be required. This test requires all the urine produced in 24 hours to be collected in a container supplied by the laboratory. The container may have special preservatives in it. Because the normal values for this test are based on an exact 24-hour collection, it is important to follow directions for urine collection carefully. Measurements of calcium and *hydroxyproline* may be made on the sample. The 24-hour urine calcium level is important in patients taking vitamin D supplements because an excess urinary calcium can cause kidney stones. Urinary hydroxyproline, which reflects the rate of bone remodeling, is usually normal in osteoporosis but may be elevated in other forms of metabolic bone disease such as hyperthyroidism and osteomalacia. Urinary hydroxyproline levels are influenced by gelatin in the diet, so a special gelatin-free diet is ordinarily consumed for several days before, and including the day of, the urine collection. A urine electrophoresis may be performed if there is proteinuria.

The Bone Scan

Many patients confuse densitometry with a bone scan. The bone scan is not useful in the diagnosis of osteoporosis, but it may be ordered by your physician to exclude other types of bone disease. In this procedure, a bone-seeking chemical that is attached to a radioactive material is injected into a vein. Wherever there is new bone being formed, there will be a greater accumulation of the radioactive material. A counter for detecting radioactivity passes over the body, and an image of the skeleton is constructed. Increased radioactivity appears in the image as "hot spots." In areas when there have been recent compression fractures there will be new bone formation and hot spots on the bone scan.

X Ray

An X-ray image is not useful in quantifying the amount of bone mineral but is necessary in making a diagnosis of osteoporosis and in excluding other forms of bone disease. There are two types of changes in the spine that suggest a diagnosis of osteoporosis: *radiolucency* and changes in shape. Very frequently a radiologist will diagnose osteoporosis on the basis of increased radiolucency (it appears that there is less bone to stop the transmission of X rays through the bone to the X-ray film). I have heard patients tell me that radiologists told them they had the bones of someone 20 years older on the basis of X-ray film that looked less dense. Unfortunately, increased radiolucency can be caused by diseases other than osteoporosis such as multiple myeloma, overactivity of the thyroid or parathyroid, and osteomalacia. In addition, increased radiolucency is not an objective finding. One radiologist may read the films as normal and another as abnormal. Again, this is not an accurate measure of bone density. The apparent density on the film may be affected by breathing and technical matters such as the distance of the patient from the X-ray tube.

Decreased density may result in the disks pushing into the vertebrae, resulting in the vertebral margins being concave instead of horizontal. Wedging is another type of deformity. Because the back muscles and the neural arch provide support for the posterior (back) surface of the vertebrae, the anterior (front) surface becomes compressed. As discussed previously, a vertebral compression or crush fracture is said to be present when there is loss of height of the posterior and usually also of the anterior portion of the vertebra.

The Bone Biopsy

Most physicians do not perform a bone biopsy on every patient with osteoporosis. Others point out that the only certain way to exclude other forms of metabolic bone disease, such as osteomalacia, is by examining sections of bone under a microscope. Because osteomalacia is relatively uncommon in the United States, a bone biopsy is performed only when another form of bone disease is suspected. Thus, if there is anything unusual about the patient clinically (e.g., young age, pain over the entire spine, or muscle weakness), biochemically (e.g., high level of alkaline phosphatase), or radiographically (e.g., X-ray signs of osteomalacia), a bone biopsy is performed.

Metabolic bone disease means that the entire skeleton is affected. This concept led to the idea that a single bone sample should reflect what is occurring in the rest of the skeleton. In a general sense, this is true. The site usually selected from the bone biopsy is the anterior iliac crest. The sample of bone is processed using special techniques to slice the bone so that it may be studied with a microscope. The sample is a core of bone that contains the outer and inner cortices (surfaces) of the site biopsied as well as the trabecular bone between the cortices.

Bone biopsies are usually performed on an outpatient basis under local anesthesia. A tranquilizer such as Valium or Vistaril may be given before the procedure begins. The skin over the iliac crest is washed and an antiseptic solution applied. A local anesthetic is used (similar to what is used when a dentist drills). After that, only pressure is felt. The surgeon makes an incision, presses a special instrument through the bone, and removes a core of bone. The incision is then closed. A bandage is placed over the incision, and the patient may go home. Pain medication (such as Percodan) may be needed for 1 to 3 days, but almost all patients are walking by the first day after the biopsy. Within a week, the sutures are removed, and the patient has no symptoms.

Examination of the biopsy under a microscope provides much information. In osteoporosis, bone volume is reduced (i.e., there is less bone per unit volume). In osteomalacia, special stains show that the osteoid (unmineralized bone) is increased in width and in the amount of trabecular surfaces it covers. Another abnormality in osteomalacia is detected by *double tetracycline labeling*. This is a technique whereby the rate of bone formation can be detected accurately. Tetracycline (a broad-spectrum antibiotic) binds to newly deposited bone and, when examined under a fluorescent microscope, may be seen as a yellow or an orange band. Before the biopsy, two courses of tetracycline are given orally (3 days each) 14 days apart. This appears as two parallel bands. The distance between the two bands is measured and divided by the time between the two tetracycline courses. Thus, if the average distance between the two lines is 14 micrometers and the time is 14 days, the rate of mineralization is 1 micrometer per day.

Microradiographs are also prepared of the bone sections. These are X rays of the bone section that are examined under a microscope. From these pictures, the percentage of bone surface that is occupied by resorption and formation activities can be determined. Counts of the number of osteoclasts and osteoblasts may also be made. The histology of bone in osteoporosis has led to a new classification of osteoporosis based on biopsy where the activity is classified as inactive (low turnover), normal, or active (high turnover).

Some centers are individualizing treatment, choosing drug therapy on the basis of whether there is high or low bone remodeling, but this approach to treatment is still under investigation.

Endometrial Biopsy

Estrogen replacement therapy (without progestins) in the prevention and treatment of osteoporosis requires periodic sampling of the endometrial tissue (lining of the womb). Endometrial biopsy involves scraping a sample of endometrial tissue for analysis by a pathologist. The biopsy is usually performed in a physician's office or in an outpatient gynecological facility. Endometrial biopsy is similar to a Pap smear in that the woman is in the same position on the examining table and similar instruments are used. Although some physicians employ a local anesthetic, often no anesthesia is necessary. Some women experience mild cramping during the procedure.

Following the biopsy, there may be minimal vaginal bleeding (staining) for several days. Some women experience uterine cramping, which can be relieved by taking mild pain-relieving medication (e.g., Tylenol) every 4 hours as needed. Following this procedure, you should notify your gynecologist if the staining becomes heavy bleeding, the bleeding continues for longer than 2 weeks, or severe or noncramping pain occurs.

SUMMARY

X rays are only a crude measurement of bone mass; health care professionals use them to diagnose osteoporosis by the presence of compression fractures. Techniques used to assess bone mass include single-photon absorptiometry of the radius, dual-photon absorptiometry and quantitative digital radiography of the lumbar spine and femur, and CAT scans of the spine. Physicians use these measurements to single out menopausal women who are at high risk for osteoporosis and to evaluate the response to drug treatment of women who already have the disease. All women should have an osteoporosis risk assessment at the time of menopause. In addition, they should address the risk factors of inactivity, poor diet, cigarette smoking, and excessive alcohol intake at this time. Those women with a history of several risk factors should be given the choice of estrogen replacement therapy. There is no point in measuring bone mineral in women who won't or can't take estrogens. Although it is unlikely that insurance companies will pay for risk assessment with bone densitometry, finding low bone density will convince many women to take estrogens, and an average or above-average value would be reassuring in such cases. Currently, dual-photon absorptiometry or quantitative digital radiography of the spine is preferred for risk assessment, but the femur may become the preferred testing site in the future.

Once a woman has been determined to have osteoporosis, the physician should conduct a variety of tests to exclude the possibility that the disease is being caused by another condition. For example, the doctor will request a bone biopsy if he or she suspects another metabolic bone disease. Bone densitometry may be used to follow the osteoporotic woman's response to various medications. Chapters 10 and 11 discuss treatment strategies for the woman with osteoporosis.

10 CHAPTER

Rehabilitative Treatment Strategies

It is exasperating to those of us who know better that patients with osteoporosis continue to be told that nothing can be done for them. In reality, most women who have suffered a compression fracture can be restored to a productive and comfortable life. Like many illnesses, osteoporosis can't be cured, but it can be treated.

REHABILITATION GOALS FOR OSTEOPOROSIS

For people with osteoporosis, the goals of treatment are not to cure, but to rehabilitate, that is, to restore their body's useful function and their own sense of well-being. The following are the specific goals of rehabilitation:

- To restore a positive outlook on life
- To increase physical activity
- To restore independence
- To allow sleep and improve appetite through treatment of depression
- To relieve pain
- To stop narcotic use
- To restore muscle mass
- To avoid fractures
- To improve posture
- To increase bone mass

This chapter discusses the treatment of a vertebral crush fracture, fracture avoidance, and the psychological adjustment to osteoporosis. Your attitude is the single most important factor in determining how well you recover from an osteoporotic fracture. Osteoporotic fractures heal normally. Although suffering a fracture represents a crisis, every crisis presents new opportunities. Those who adjust will find new opportunities to improve their health habits.

TREATMENT IMMEDIATELY FOLLOWING VERTEBRAL FRACTURE

Wedge fractures of the spine may go unnoticed. An older woman may simply observe that she has become shorter and more round-shouldered. It is unusual to have your height measured in adult life, so many osteoporotic women are shocked when we do measure them because they did not realize the extent of their reduction in height. Other osteoporotic fractures usually attract immediate attention because of severe pain. The woman who fell and now lies on the floor with pain in her hip and her leg rotated outward will get immediate attention. The woman who broke her fall with an outstretched hand will also have pain and deformity in the wrist and will be diagnosed promptly. The affectionate hug from a grand-child that is followed by pain in the chest that increases when you breathe in and cough will probably result in an X ray and a diagno-sis of a fractured rib.

The back pain that results from a crush fracture will also usually attract immediate attention but may be more difficult to diagnose. The pain is sudden and severe and may not be confined to the back but may travel around the rib cage (on one side or both) and to the front of the chest or the abdomen, depending on whether the in-volved vertebra is in the thoracic or the lumbar spine. Occasionally, the pain seems worse in the front of the body or even the flank. Pain from osteoporotic fractures may be confused with heart attack, kid-ney stones, gallbladder attack, pancreatitis, dissecting aneurysm, and shingles. The astute physician will obtain an X ray of the spine and will dismiss these other conditions.

Common situations in which women have developed vertebral crush fractures include tucking the bedspread under the mattress, lifting a roast out of the oven, and trying to open a stuck window or garage door. These stresses can be so severe on the osteoporotic spine that individual vertebrae become compressed. As a result, the vertebra is now more dense and may be more resistant to the compressive forces that are normally inflicted on the spine. Indeed, even if osteoporosis is not treated, another fracture of the spine will probably not occur for several years because the spine has become more dense.

Following a compression fracture, severe pain persists for 3 to 6 weeks while the vertebra heals. During the first 3 weeks, most patients remain in bed much of the time and are given narcotics to relieve the pain. Narcotic medications cause constipation, and straining to have a bowel movement can cause excruciating back pain. Therefore, it is important to keep the stools soft with medication and plenty of fluids. A hard mattress with a sheepskin cover or foam rubber "egg crate" (to avoid pressure sores) is used. The patient is permitted to stay in whatever position is most comfortable, even on the side with support from a pillow. If the patient cannot find a comfortable position in bed, a recommended one is to have the patient lie on her back with her knees flexed with a thin pillow to support the head and regular-sized pillows placed below the knees (to keep them flexed) and between the legs. Attempts to relieve pain can be made by relaxing the muscles around the spine. Heat is applied through an infrared lamp, and gentle massage is used.

After about 2 or 3 weeks, most patients can get up to go to the bathroom and nonnarcotic painkillers can be substituted. It may be necessary to use a walker at first. Gradually, activity can be increased to the prefracture level (or greater). Exercising in a heated pool may be useful, or a walking program can be started (see the exercise program outlined in chapter 8) under the guidance of a physician or *physical therapist*. Pain medication may be reduced or eliminated. Like any fracture, the fracture of a vertebra takes time to heal. After it has healed, there may be no further pain unless another fracture occurs. Although recovery time from a crush fracture will vary from person to person, most women are completely recovered within 6 to 8 weeks.

REHABILITATIVE TREATMENT OF VERTEBRAL FRACTURES

As much as 1 to 8 inches of height is lost as a result of vertebral compression fractures. This is not as disturbing to most women as are the compensatory changes in posture. A collapsed vertebrae is collapsed forever. As a result of thoracic fractures, *kyphosis* (hunchback), or curvature of the upper spine, occurs. The spine is shortened so that the arms are disproportionately longer than the trunk.

Also, the abdomen has less space for its intestinal contents and abdominal organs, and a potbelly, or protuberant abdomen, develops. The hips are flexed to maintain balance, and many women walk with the feet spaced further apart and take slower steps. Part of the change in posture is also due to muscle atrophy (loss of muscle tissue) from disuse. Much of the chronic pain in osteoporosis is due to changes in the configuration of the spine.

Improving Posture

If you maintain the kyphotic posture that naturally follows a compression fracture, the muscles and ligaments around the spine will become shortened and you will not be able to stand erect. Exercises that pinch the shoulders together and the stand-tall exercise (chapter 8) are useful in combating kyphosis. Other important postural exercises are the wall stretch and deep breathing. As a result of shortening of the spine, the lower rib cage may rub against the brim of the pelvis, resulting in pain of the lower ribs. This can be overcome by stretching exercises. These exercises also help reduce pain caused by muscle spasm. Indeed, if your back muscles start aching during the day, try the stand-tall exercise for relief.

Make a conscious effort to avoid stooping. Think about your posture throughout the day. Keep your head high with your chin pulled in and your shoulder blades pinched in toward each other. Practice walking in this manner with a pillow on your head for a few minutes several times a day. If you are standing for a long time, rest one foot on a stool for a while and then switch weight to the other foot.

When you are sitting, keep a pillow or a rolled towel in the small of your back. Increase the thickness of the headrest in your car to support your neck. Bring your desk toward you and adjust the height of your chair so you do not have to stoop when doing paperwork or when typing. If you have been sitting for a while and feel uncomfortable, take a break and do the wall-arch exercise (chapter 8).

When lying down or sleeping, it is preferable to be on your back. You may be more comfortable with a towel roll under your back, and you may need two pillows to support your neck. If you sleep comfortably only on your side, try not to assume the fetal position, but you may bend your knees slightly.

Braces, Corsets, and Jackets

Spinal devices (orthoses) have a limited role in rehabilitating the victim of a vertebral crush fracture. Spinal orthoses should be considered as temporary devices that can be discarded following a program of physical therapy. The purposes of spinal bracing are to

- decrease pain,
- protect against any further injury, and
- prevent or help correct the deformity that follows a vertebral fracture.

Braces accomplish these goals by providing trunk support, limiting motion, and realigning the vertebrae, but their effectiveness is usually limited. Braces neither completely immobilize nor realign the spine. Rather, by applying pressure on bone, they produce enough discomfort to remind the patient to limit motion or to maintain posture. Braces and corsets supply support to the spine by pressing (usually uncomfortably) on the abdomen. This increases the pressure on the abdomen and decreases the pressure on the lumbar spine.

Lumbosacral corsets are usually made of canvas with rigid steel backs and adjustable lacing on the side or back. The most commonly used lumbosacral rigid brace is the chair-back brace. This brace controls extension, flexion, and motion from side to side. Plastic lumbar supports that are molded to the shape of the lumbar spine and that fit into a pouch in a corset are also available. Molded jackets may be made of plaster or preferably of thermoplastic and can be fitted to provide uniform pressure and support to the trunk. Temporary use of these devices allows a patient with a recent spinal fracture to get out of bed and walk around sooner.

Thoracolumbar corsets primarily provide abdominal support but also serve as reminders to maintain posture. There are two types of thoracolumbar braces: the Taylor brace and molded jackets. The Taylor brace limits thoracic motion by tightening the straps that are wrapped around the shoulders so tight that they are painful. When the patient understandably loosens the straps, the brace becomes ineffective. A more effective thoracolumbar brace is the chair-back brace with the cow-horn or sternal pad attachments, which result in pressure being transmitted through the sternum and ribs to the spine. Spinal support and limitation of spinal motion are provided by pressure in other areas.

Effective bracing can produce discomfort, and there are other potential disadvantages to using them for a prolonged period of time. Muscle weakness and atrophy may occur because of the decreased need for activity of the trunk muscles. A greater effort must be made to carry out activities when wearing a brace, and this may be undesirable in elderly patients with heart or lung disease. Some women become psychologically dependent on orthoses even though they do not benefit from wearing the device. Remember that bracing, if needed, should usually be used for only a few months after a fracture. They are usually prescribed only for the woman who is unable to get out of bed without severe pain several weeks after sustaining a crush fracture and are ordinarily discarded within a few months.

AVOIDING FUTURE VERTEBRAL FRACTURES

A major objective after recovering from a fracture is to avoid another fracture. Remember that there are two factors that determine your risk for fracture: the strength of the skeleton and the forces applied to the skeleton. The woman who develops a fractured vertebra after lifting a heavy bundle or who fractures a hip after a fall had the same bone density (strength) a moment before the fracture. Prudence dictates that a woman with osteoporosis avoid situations that could lead to a fall or injury to the spine. I am always unnerved by the woman who tells me, "I have great news. I fell down the stairs yesterday and did not break any bones." I always respond with, "Please, please try to avoid falling. The next 'test' may not be successful." Be careful at family gatherings where an affectionate hug may result in a fractured rib. Review the tips on how to avoid injury that were discussed in chapter 4.

PSYCHOLOGICAL ADJUSTMENT TO OSTEOPOROSIS AND FRACTURES

There are also some common psychological problems that occur in women who have suffered osteoporotic fractures. Pain produces not only a lack of mobility but also insomnia. It further hinders the ability of osteoporotic women to cope with their illness. *Analgesics* (painkillers) can make one less alert. Some patients actually become dependent on narcotic analgesics. Appropriate treatment of pain is essential in the management of osteoporosis and will be discussed in chapter 11.

A Grieving Process

A grieving process for the losses from osteoporosis (similar to that following the death of a loved one) frequently follows the occurrence of a crush fracture. This process may start with shock, disbelief, and anger. Intense sadness may follow as well as an unwillingness to accept what has happened. The grieving process should be understood by friends and family members and treated with understanding and compassion. It should last only several weeks or months. A successful grief reaction eventually results in accepting the realities that osteoporosis has imposed, in a renewed sense of energy, and in a new interest in minimizing disability and getting on with life. If the feelings of blueness persist after several months or there is a very deep sense of despondency, a physician should be consulted. Depression may be successfully treated with counseling and *antidepressant* medication.

Fear of Future Fractures

After recovering from a fracture, some patients become disabled by the fear of incurring another fracture. I remember an osteoporotic woman who took a long time to walk down the corridor to the examining room and who required assistance to sit on the examining table. After commenting sympathetically that she must be in a great deal of pain, I was astounded to find that at the time she had no pain whatsoever. However, she was afraid that a slight movement in the wrong direction would result in another compression fracture. This woman now leads an active life and through education has overcome her fear of fracture.

Sexual Adjustment

Related to the fear of fracture is the fear of injury during sexual relations. Very often it is the partner of the osteoporotic woman who is afraid that he will injure his wife. Unfortunately, very few women discuss this concern openly with their physician. As a result, many women have deprived themselves and their husbands of years of sexual pleasure. If your physician does not discuss sexual relations, ask him about it when you discuss which physical activities should be avoided.

There is no reason why an osteoporotic woman cannot have an active and fulfilling sex life. As with physical exercise, there should be neither active flexion of the spine nor undue force on the ribs during sexual intercourse. The commonly used positions during sexual intercourse are safe, particularly with a gentle, caring partner. The crossover position is particularly comfortable. Perhaps this is the opportunity to read a sex education manual and to attempt to enhance your sexuality. Perhaps it is even more important to realize that there is much more to sexuality than the act of sexual intercourse. The pleasure of being held and caressed by someone who loves you is precious even when pain may make the act of sexual intercourse undesirable.

Fear of Dependency

One of the greatest fears of osteoporotic women is that they will become dependent on their spouse or children. Worse yet is the fear of total disability and life in a nursing home. Consider the statement of Mrs. Z: "I hate to be a burden to my children. My husband has been sick with cancer, and he needs me to take care of him. I won't be able to help him anymore. I'm very upset at even temporarily living with my daughter—she has her own problems. Even if I get better I will have to move out of my home into an apartment and put my husband into a nursing home. Besides, my children have always depended on me. Now, they are treating me as though I am a child and trying to tell me what is best for me and my husband. Worse yet, I may become a financial burden to my children." Physicians should try to be sensitive to concerns such as these and should try to discuss them with patients as any other medical matter would be discussed.

Accept the love and care that your family willingly gives you. If you have a caring family, it is only because of the love and care you give to them. Allow your family to help you recover. Seek medical care and gradually increase your physical activity. You may have to accept temporary help to prevent permanent disability. Remember, osteoporosis can be successfully treated.

Altered Body Image

The change in body shape that results from compression fractures is disturbing to many women. It is common to hear, "How could this have happened to me? I had such a nice figure. It seems as though I have become stooped and old almost overnight. I can't stand to look in a mirror at how bent over I have become. My clothes don't fit me anymore. You tell me to use a cane but I don't want to look old. I resent people offering to help me around. I am so ashamed that this has happened to me."

Some women avoid public places and old acquaintances. They stay at home, avoid their friends, and become depressed. Other women have a more positive outlook. They know that there is much more to being an attractive woman than simply having an attractive figure. They take the opportunity to develop other personal assets. They also develop even greater attention to dress and other aspects of personal appearance such as their hairstyle and makeup. Think of your positive points. Develop them further. Practice positive self-talk. Compliment yourself. Keep working at developing greater self-confidence. Those women who feel good about themselves recover best from osteoporosis.

The use of corsets, shoulder straps, and exercise may improve your appearance. There is currently no way to restore the pre-fracture height of a vertebra. Thus, the reasons for the change in the body's appearance should be understood and eventually accepted. Clothing should be chosen that minimizes kyphosis and that takes into consideration that the trunk has shortened whereas the extremities have stayed the same size. Table 10.1 provides fashion tips for the osteoporotic woman. Custom tailoring is a good idea. It is possible to appear quite attractive if special attention is paid to selection of clothing.

Table 10.1   Fashion Suggestions

Problem	Suggestions
Decrease in trunk size	Pleated blouse
	Blousons
	Jacket dresses
	Long vest sweaters
	Wear blouse with hem at mid-abdomen rather than waist
Dorsal kyphosis	Gathered sleeves
	Cowl necklines
	Shawl necklines
	Dropped shoulders
Protuberant abdomen	Soft corset
	Long torso dresses
	Blouse with hem at mid-abdomen

SUMMARY

A vertebral crush fracture commonly occurs when mechanical stress is placed on the osteoporotic spine. This type of fracture is usually painful and often requires 2 to 3 weeks of bed rest before recovery begins. When the patient gets out of bed, she may need a custom-fitted, temporary spinal support. However, changes in posture may still result in continued pain because of muscle spasms. The treatment includes an adequate intake of calcium and vitamin D (400 IU daily). The patient receives instruction on exercise, posture control, and how to avoid falls and back injuries. In general, the primary goal of rehabilitating the osteoporotic woman is to restore a positive outlook on life. Treatment of pain and the use of medication to prevent further bone loss will be described in chapters 11 and 12.

11 CHAPTER

Treatment of Pain From Osteoporosis

Fortunately, most women with osteoporosis don't have chronic, or persistent, pain. After a fractured vertebra heals, pain is usually no longer a problem. However, in some osteoporotic women, pain persists and is disabling. This chapter is specifically for these women, their health professionals, and their families. It discusses the causes of chronic pain, lists various treatment strategies for pain associated with osteoporotic fractures, and addresses the use of pain clinics as one possible form of therapy.

THE CAUSES OF CHRONIC PAIN

If pain persists beyond the time that it would be expected for a vertebral fracture to have healed, the physician must reinvestigate and ask the following questions:

- Are there new fractures?
- Is there another cause for the pain (e.g., *herniated disk*, arthritis, scoliosis)?
- Is the pain from pull on ligaments?
- Is the pain from muscle spasms?
- Are exercises causing the pain?
- Are microfractures (tiny fractures that do not appear in X ray) occurring?
- Has the patient become dependent on narcotics?
- Is the patient depressed?
- How well does the patient tolerate pain?
- Are the lower ribs rubbing against the pelvic brim, thus causing pain?

The answers to these questions are usually not obvious. X-ray findings may be misleading. An abnormal X ray does not indicate whether the abnormal finding is the cause of pain. Some individuals have multiple abnormalities on X ray that could be associated with pain, yet they are entirely free of back pain. On the other hand, some individuals have severe back pain with no abnormalities on their X-ray films.

A MULTIPLE-FRONT APPROACH TO TREATING CHRONIC PAIN

Treatment may begin with a simultaneous attack on several fronts. A brace or support may be prescribed if the pain is due to the change in shape of the spine with associated muscle spasms. Heat and massage are also used for muscle pain. Antidepressant medication lowers the perception of pain. Exercises to improve posture and relieve ligament strain and muscle spasms can be initiated. Stretching exercise and deep breathing may reduce discomfort from the lower ribs rubbing against the pelvic brim. Medication aimed at increasing bone mass may be prescribed.

One particular type of muscle spasm is quite common after recovery from a fracture of the thoracic spine. There is an increase in *lumbar lordosis* (the curve of the lumbar spine) with associated lumbar muscle spasm and lower-back pain. This can be relieved by intermittent spinal rest. The patient is instructed to get off her feet (in bed) for 20 to 30 minutes every 3 hours. For women with lumbar pain, I usually prescribe using a fitted plastic support with an expandable front to allow the abdomen to protrude. The support is worn only when the patient is on her feet for long periods. The pain usually subsides after 3 months, and the patient may then discontinue the rest periods if she is pain free.

As with any other problem, the proper management of pain is greatly aided by understanding the underlying causes. For example, following a compression fracture of the spine, it may be necessary to use narcotic drugs for pain relief despite the small risk of drug addiction. However, after several weeks, when the patient begins to get out of bed and walk, the associated pain may be from muscle spasms rather than from the fractured vertebra. This would be better treated with heat, nonnarcotic drugs for pain relief, and perhaps a spinal corset. It is important to understand the cause of pain and to avoid narcotic addiction and chronic pain due to the *learned pain syndrome*, a condition that will be discussed later in this chapter.

It is also important to understand that pain produces emotional distress. On the other hand, the conception of patients and even of some health professionals that pain may be "imagined" is nonsense. More important, to be well you must concentrate not on pain but on your ability to behave the same way you did before you were diagnosed as having osteoporosis. Your goal should be to struggle against disability. Some methods for managing chronic pain follow.

- Drugs
- Physical therapy
- Electrical stimulation
- Acupuncture
- Hypnosis
- Biofeedback
- Behavior modification

Discussions of each of these methods follow.

USES OF DRUGS
IN PAIN TREATMENT

There are three classes of drugs that may be used to alleviate pain: narcotics, nonnarcotic analgesics ("analgesia" means relief of pain), and psychoactive drugs (medications that affect the mind).

Narcotic Drugs

Narcotic drugs should be used only for severe pain (such as a fracture) and for a short period of time because they are habit forming.

Awareness of the placebo effect should convince you that you can manage pain without the active ingredients in drugs. Most studies that are designed to prove a drug's effectiveness have one group of patients take the active drug and another, comparison group that thinks they are taking the active drug but are actually taking a placebo.

Placebos do indeed relieve pain. They provide about half the pain relief of the drug the patient believes is being taken. Thus, if the treatment group is taking aspirin, the placebo group will obtain about half the relief obtained from aspirin; if the treatment group receives a more potent narcotic, the placebo group will get greater pain relief (i.e., half the pain relief obtained from the narcotic drug). An explanation for the placebo effect has recently been found.

Placebos may cause the release of *endorphins* (chemical substances in the brain that produce analgesia) and are probably related to the way narcotics relieve pain.

Nonnarcotic Drugs

When pain is not severe, the nonsteroidal *anti-inflammatory* drugs may be prescribed. The oldest and probably the safest of these are aspirin and acetaminophen (found in Tylenol). These drugs should be taken about every 6 hours. Many of the other drugs now available were introduced as arthritis medications but later were found to have analgesic properties. Those who do not obtain relief from one drug in this group may still benefit from another drug in the group. The side effects of these drugs are similar: gastric irritation *(gastritis)* and liver, kidney, and blood toxicity. The nonsteroidal anti-inflammatory drugs (with the exception of aspirin) also tend to be expensive. Do not hesitate to take these medications if you have pain that limits your activity, but be sure to consult your physician first.

Psychoactive Drugs

Another class of drugs that are often useful, especially when used in combination with the nonsteroidal anti-inflammatory drugs, are antidepressant, or *antipsychotic*, drugs. It is not known exactly how these drugs act, but it is known that depression worsens pain. If there are symptoms of depression (e.g., crying, feeling blue, loss of appetite, lack of socialization, or loss of interest in sex) that persist beyond the normal grieving process described in chapter 10, antidepressants can relieve both pain and depression. When lecturing on osteoporosis, I like to make the statement that I have helped more women recover from osteoporosis by prescription of antidepressants than anyone ever helped with fluoride or other medications.

Antidepressant drugs are not habit forming. They are useful in the treatment of pain even in the absence of depression. However, a recent study suggests that these medications may increase the risk for hip fracture, presumably by increasing the chance of falling. Thus, use these medications cautiously.

USES OF OTHER MODALITIES FOR PAIN TREATMENT

Transcutaneous electrical nerve stimulation, or *TENS*, involves a battery-operated machine with electrodes that are placed on the skin. The impulses generated by these instruments cause the release of endorphins in the brain. Most often, the pain relief is of a relatively short duration. *Acupuncture* is another form of transcutaneous stimulation and works well. These forms of therapy are reserved for patients who do not respond to the nonsteroidal anti-inflammatory drugs, antidepressants, and exercise. Two other methods in current use are *biofeedback* and hypnosis. In biofeedback an electromyogram is used to detect muscle tension; the patient is informed of the tense muscles and learns to relax them. Hypnosis probably acts in a fashion similar to placebo by releasing endorphins.

Behavior modification is an important form of therapy for all patients with chronic pain. It is designed to change responses to pain. The three major goals of behavioral therapy are

- to eliminate reinforcers of pain behavior,
- to increase physical activity (through activity based on a quota rather than pain), and
- to eliminate drug therapy.

The techniques of behavior modification are used in most pain clinics.

One technique of behavioral therapy that you can try is relaxation breathing. When you have severe pain, lie down and close your eyes. Place one hand on the chest and the other on the abdomen and breathe deeply. You should try to breathe the way you do when you sleep, that is, abdominal breathing. The hand on your abdomen should rise and fall as you breathe, whereas the hand on your chest should barely move. Breathe slowly in (count to 4) and out (count to 5).

Another technique to reduce pain involves the use of *imagery*. There are four imagery techniques:

- Concentrate on the pain and transform it into a fantasy object, such as a bird, and allow it to leave the body.
- Imagine a pleasant situation that is incompatible with pain, such as ocean waves or walking through the woods.

- Imagine that the sensation is not pain but rather numbness.
- Practice distraction by doing arithmetic or analyzing separate musical parts as you listen to the recording of a concerto or symphony.

The treatment of pain due to fracture is somewhat different than the treatment of pain due to muscle spasm, which will be discussed next.

TREATMENT OF PAIN DUE TO MUSCLE SPASMS

There are some other suggestions that may help reduce pain due to muscle spasms. Relaxation techniques may be helpful. Moist heat, a heating pad, or even a gentle rubdown with Ben-Gay may give you relief. When your back is troublesome, you may find that getting off your feet (in bed or on a couch) for 10 minutes every few hours will enable you to do more when you are up. A cushion should be placed behind the small of the back when you are sitting or riding in a car. Raise the height of your typewriter or desk. Kitchen counters may be too high for you now. Consider the possibility of new custom kitchen cabinets.

Also, remember that aspirin or Tylenol are not habit forming. If you have mild pain, take one of these medications. Some women refuse to take analgesics until their back pain is severe. By that time, though, these safer medications will probably not help. Do not place a positive moral value on pain. Being productive is preferable to bearing pain.

WHO SHOULD ATTEND A PAIN CLINIC?

Who should attend a pain clinic? An easy answer is all those with pain that is disabling and that has not responded to treatment by a physician. Certainly patients with learned pain syndrome could benefit from attending a pain clinic. These are patients who are addicted to narcotics or overly dependent on physicians, family, or friends. They feel helpless and are unable to carry out normal social functions. They are often homebound. Subconsciously, they have learned to behave in a sick, dependent role. Through behavior modification techniques, they can learn healthy behavior. If your physician suggests that you attend a pain clinic, have an open mind. The reward may be a return to self-reliance and a more normal life.

SUMMARY

Chronic pain usually is not a problem for osteoporotic women. When pain does persist after a vertebral fracture heals, the physician should look for other possible causes of the pain. If he or she can identify the cause, then pain management is specific. Physicians often treat pain with multiple, simultaneous approaches that may include analgesic medication, antidepressants, bracing, and specific exercises. Muscle spasms are sometimes treated with heat and massage. Narcotics should be avoided except immediately following a fracture. Some patients engage in TENS, hypnosis, accupuncture, and biofeedback to deal with chronic pain, and others are referred to a pain clinic. In several cases, the treatment strategy employed will depend on the individual involved.

12 CHAPTER

Drug Therapy for Osteoporosis

You can appreciate the difficulty in reducing the risk for future fractures when you consider the goals of osteoporotic therapy. A fracture develops primarily because of low bone mass. If the normal loss of bone that occurs with aging is reversed, bone mass stays the same as before treatment, and the risk for fracture remains the same (see Figure 12.1). This is certainly preferable to the additional bone loss that would result from avoiding treatment, and the even greater subsequent risk for fracture. However, the ideal treatment for osteoporosis would actually *increase* bone mass. This involves not only reversing the aging process of bone, but also returning to the phase of bone growth that normally occurs during childhood and the childbearing age. To add to this difficulty, we normally lose bone mass at the rate of 1% to 1.5% per year, but a woman with osteoporotic fractures has almost 20% less bone than a woman of the same age with no osteoporotic fractures. In this case, restoring a strong skeleton might require treatment for 15 to 20 years. The treatment of osteoporosis is a long-term process.

Despite these difficulties, the outlook for drug treatment in osteoporosis has become brighter in the past several years. *Quantitative* bone-mass measurements have shown that bone mass can be increased in women with osteoporosis. A decade ago, most researchers didn't believe that this would ever be possible. Furthermore, several studies have shown that we can reduce the number of subsequent fractures by treating osteoporosis with drugs. This chapter discusses some of these drugs in detail.

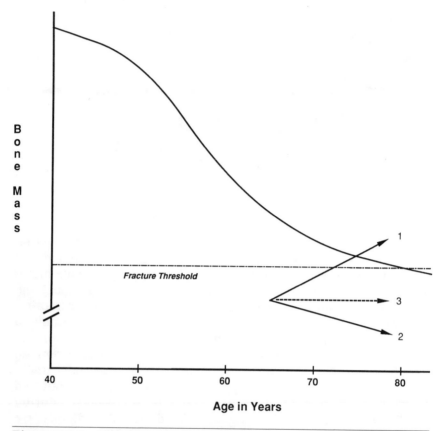

Figure 12.1   The theoretically ideal treatment would increase bone mass above the fracture threshold (line 1) rather than only preventing further bone loss (line 3). If no other treatment were given bone loss would continue (line 2).

CHARACTERISTICS OF IDEAL DRUG THERAPY

The purpose of antiosteoporotic drug treatment is to reduce the likelihood of future fractures by increasing bone mass. It is useful to consider the characteristics of an "ideal" form of medication for treatment of osteoporosis:

- The drug should be safe.
- The drug should increase bone mass to such a level that there is no further risk for fracture.

- The new bone formed should be architecturally sound; that is, it should be normal bone in composition and structure.
- The medication should be easy to take and readily accepted by patients.

It should be emphasized that, although this may change in the near future, drugs currently labeled as effective in the treatment of osteoporosis by the FDA include only estrogen and salmon calcitonin.

CLASSIFICATION OF NEW DRUG TREATMENTS

Because all drugs have side effects, it is always important to weigh the risks of drug treatment against the anticipated benefits. The exciting news is that bone loss can be prevented with FDA-approved drug therapy using calcitonin or estrogens. Furthermore, new treatments designed to increase bone mass are currently being investigated. A classification of the mechanism of action of these drugs follows.

Classification
of Treatment Mechanisms

Inhibitors (Reduce bone remodeling)

- Calcium
- Estrogen
- Testosterone
- Progesterone
- Anabolic steroids
- Calcitonin
- Diphosphonates

Activators (Increase bone formation)

- Fluoride
- Growth hormone
- Phosphates
- Low-dose parathyroid hormone

(Cont.)

Classification of Treatment Mechanisms (Continued)

Combination Therapy (Increases bone formation; decreases remodeling)

Concurrent use of a medication that stimulates bone formation with one that decreases bone resorption

Sequential Therapy (Increases bone formation; decreases remodeling)

Use of activator drugs for several months, followed by the use of inhibitor drugs, followed by a period of no drug treatment and then repetition of the sequence.

Calcium Absorption (Stimulates the absorption of calcium)

- Ergocalciferol
- Calcitriol
- Other forms of vitamin D

Remember that all drugs have side effects and that prescription of any of these FDA-approved drugs should be considered carefully.

DRUGS THAT REDUCE
BONE RESORPTION

Calcium supplementation is often ignored in a discussion of the treatment of osteoporosis. It is clear that 1,000 to 1,500 milligrams of calcium per day does not prevent bone loss in women with osteoporosis. However, it is generally accepted that every patient with osteoporosis should have a total daily intake of 1,000 to 1,500 milligrams of calcium. It would be more accurate to refer to taking this amount of calcium as repletion rather than supplementation of the diet.

Implementing Calcium Supplementation

Recent studies suggest that calcium supplements in large amounts may help prevent bone loss in women with postmenopausal osteoporosis. This protective effect has been observed with bone-density measurements of cortical rather than trabecular bone. The total amount of calcium intake in these studies exceeded 2,000 to 2,500 milligrams of elemental calcium per day. Calcium in these doses should be considered a medication. Discuss this with your physician.

Calcium supplementation should definitely be used in combination with all other drug treatment regimens. If a drug acts to decrease the amount of bone that is resorbed, then it is possible to get a secondary increase in parathyroid hormone secretion. This might then increase bone resorption and produce bone loss, which can be prevented by obtaining an adequate amount of calcium. Moreover, if a drug produces new bone, then there must be an adequate amount of calcium present so that the bone will be normally mineralized. Thus, all forms of treatment should be accompanied by an adequate calcium intake either by diet or by supplementation.

Gonadal Steroids

One of the oldest treatments for osteoporosis is therapy with gonadal steroids (estrogen and androgens) (Albright, 1947).

Estrogen

Generally, women within 10 to 15 years of menopause are treated with estrogen (most physicians prefer treatment with calcitonin in older women). It is recommended that patients who take estrogen have the same type of management as is recommended for estrogen-replacement therapy after menopause. Thus, they should also take progestins and have regular physical exams, including pelvic and breast exams, measurement of blood pressure, Pap smears, and perhaps endometrial sampling.

There is a common misunderstanding about the decrease in effectiveness of estrogens when they are given more than 6 years after menopause. Estrogens do continue to inhibit bone loss in older women. However, if a woman lost 10% of her premenopausal bone mass between the ages of 50 and 56 and another 10% in the ensuing decade, it is clear that starting estrogen at age 66 instead of 50 cannot replace the 20% reduction of bone mass.

Androgens

The effectiveness of androgens or *anabolic steroids*, is more controversial. Anabolic steroids are drugs that have the biochemical effects of testosterone (male hormone) with less of the masculinizing effects. Masculinizing effects include growth of facial hair, deepening of the voice, and acne. There are a variety of anabolic steroids available. Investigators at the University of Washington (Chesnut, Nelp, & Baylink, 1977) found that anabolic steroids increase bone mass. At Brookhaven National Laboratory (Aloia, Kapoor, Vaswani, & Cohn, 1981) we studied an anabolic steroid and were unable to demonstrate any benefit in terms of changes in bone mass. Moreover, we could easily tell which patients were taking the anabolic steroid and which received a placebo because of the evident masculinizing effects. These drugs are not approved for use in the treatment of osteoporosis.

Calcitonin

Early studies using calcitonin did not employ calcium supplementation. Therefore, we would now predict that there was a secondary increase in parathyroid hormone and that bone was lost. More recent studies in which calcium supplementation was used have demonstrated that there is an increase in bone mass following the treatment of osteoporosis with calcitonin (Mazzuoli et al., 1986). This drug has been used in Europe for many years and has been approved for use by the FDA for treating osteoporosis. It is the safest drug available for this purpose, but its major disadvantage is that it currently has to be given by injection. However, just as our patients with diabetes have learned to give themselves injections, so our patients with osteoporosis have mastered this skill easily.

Calcitonin is remarkably free of serious side effects. I have used this drug in research projects and then in practice since 1970 and have never observed a serious complication. However, symptoms of gastrointestinal upset and flushing may occur in as many as 10% to 20% of patients. Some patients experience increased urinary frequency.

There is an additional advantage of calcitonin therapy in that it has a mild analgesic effect, thus giving patients the added benefit of a reduction in pain. A nasal spray is being tested for delivery of calcitonin so that injections may not be needed in the future. Instructions for giving injections of calcitonin are given in Appendix 12.A to this chapter. These instructions with photos are an excellent addition to patient instruction in the home use of calcitonin. Salmon calcitonin (Calcimar) is the drug that is currently used for treating osteoporosis. Human calcitonin has been recently released in the United States, but it has not yet been approved by the FDA for use in treating osteoporosis.

Diphosphonates are another class of drugs that inhibit bone resorption. They are currently used in the treatment of another bone disease called Pagets' disease. Initial studies with this medication were disappointing, and, like therapy with fluoride, diphosphonates have the potential to produce an abnormal bone structure. However, recent research suggests that diphosphonates should be studied further and may be useful in treating osteoporosis.

DRUGS THAT INCREASE BONE FORMATION

Sodium fluoride is the only drug in widespread use that stimulates bone formation. It is not currently approved for use by the FDA. Despite having been available for a number of years, the use of sodium fluoride in the treatment of osteoporosis is still considered investigational. The Mayo Clinic has published information that suggests that fluoride may reduce the occurrence of spinal fractures in osteoporotic patients (Riggs, Seeman, Hodgson, Taves, & O'Fallon, 1982). This group is currently participating in a multi-centered clinical trial to determine the safety and efficacy of fluoride. This study should be completed soon. It is important to realize that the dosage of fluoride used to treat osteoporosis is 45 times the amount that is used to prevent dental cavities. This is a very large dose and is potentially toxic. Moreover, excessive fluoride can cause a type of bone disease called fluorosis, which increases susceptibility to fractures. Frequent side effects of fluoride use include gastrointestinal upset and joint pain.

Some preliminary results from the Mayo Clinic were reported at a research meeting in Denmark in late 1987. Fluoride treatment increased bone density of the spine but not of the whole skeleton. There is concern that fluoride treatment may increase trabecular bone while decreasing cortical bone. Moreover, fluoride therapy was associated with the development of stress fractures. It is evident that fluoride treatment should be confined to research centers until the risk-benefit ratio of fluoride is known.

The Winthrop-Brookhaven research group (Aloia et al., 1976) has studied the use of growth hormone in the treatment of osteoporosis, and others (Reeve et al., 1980) have studied the use of a low dose of parathyroid hormone. These forms of therapy do not appear to produce an increase in bone mass. It is unlikely that either growth hormone or parathyroid hormone when used alone will be beneficial to patients with osteoporosis.

COMBINATION DRUG THERAPY

A number of studies suggest that treatment with drugs that decrease bone resorption do not produce a sustained increase in bone mass. Medication that reduces the number of remodeling units will prevent bone loss, but will not produce a continuing increase in bone mass. To accomplish this objective, bone formation must be increased to a level above that of bone resorption. Several investigators have therefore developed the concept of combination therapy for osteoporosis. In this scheme of treatment, a drug is given to reduce bone resorption simultaneously with a drug that increases bone formation. Thus, both sides of the bone-remodeling unit are attacked at the same time.

As with all other treatment regimens, calcium supplements are also taken. Of the drugs that we have thus far studied at Brookhaven National Laboratory, the highest increase in bone mass we have observed is with patients who were treated with a combination of fluoride, estrogen, and calcium (Aloia, Zanzi, Vaswani, Ellis, & Cohn, 1982). It is important to note that Mayo Clinic researchers have also observed the greatest reduction in fracture rate in patients who were treated with this combination (Riggs, Wahner, et al., 1982). Because these studies were not definitive and because the risk-benefit ratios are not totally known, this form of therapy is not generally recommended at this time. Other combinations have proven less successful. For example, the Winthrop-Brookhaven research group (Aloia, Vaswani, Kapoor, Yeh, & Cohn, 1985) has treated patients with a combination of growth hormone, calcitonin, and calcium and found no advantage over treatment with either calcitonin or calcium alone.

SEQUENTIAL DRUG THERAPY

The order of the normal bone-cell cycle has resulted in a proposal that osteoporosis may be treated successfully with sequential, or coherence, therapy (Frost, 1979). In this scheme patients are first given an agent that increases bone remodeling. It is theoretically possible to produce changes of considerable magnitude in skeletal mass by dramatically increasing the number of remodeling units. This is followed by treatment with an agent that inhibits bone resorption. The next phase of the treatment cycle is a rest period during which time new bone is laid down by osteoblasts. This sequence is repeated indefinitely. Although this is an exciting proposal for an effective means to increase bone mass continuously, there is insufficient information to determine whether this form of treatment will be successful.

DRUGS THAT INCREASE CALCIUM ABSORPTION

As discussed earlier, one of the major effects of vitamin D is its ability to increase calcium absorption. A number of elderly people have low levels of vitamin D probably as a result not only of diet but also of reduced exposure to sunshine. Moreover, as one grows older, it is increasingly difficult for the kidneys to form the active metabolite of vitamin D (i.e., calcitriol). There is controversy as to which form of vitamin D is best in attempting to increase calcium absorption. The active metabolites of vitamin D have a shorter half-life; that is, they are present in the body for a shorter period of time. Therefore, they have the advantage that, if there is a vitamin D overdose, their effects would last for a shorter period of time. Each form of vitamin D will increase calcium absorption in the intestine. An excessive amount of any of these forms will also produce further bone loss and may result in kidney stones and high blood calcium.

Calcitriol may prevent bone loss. However, the risks involved for renal function in order to achieve high blood levels of calcitriol make it unlikely that treatment with calcitriol will be useful. Future studies are planned using a form of calcitriol that is not taken orally (Aloia, Vaswani, Yeh, Yasumura, & Cohn, 1988).

WHO SHOULD UNDERGO DRUG THERAPY?

The choice of whether to receive drug therapy and of which drugs to take should be an informed choice made with the help of your physician. Treatment must be specific to each patient, and special consideration must be given to each individual's risk. For example, a woman who had breast cancer in the past might not be given estrogen. She could obtain the same effect on the skeleton, however, with calcitonin and calcium supplements.

There must also be a realistic appreciation of the limitations of drug therapy for osteoporosis. The objective is long term, that is, to reduce future risk for fracture by preventing further bone loss (or, ideally, increasing bone mass). Women with recent crush fractures might want to begin therapy immediately because of their desire for pain relief and increased activity. It is difficult for them to accept that these goals are accomplished by the passage of time, exercise, and analgesics. On the other hand, women who have recovered from their last fracture often want to discontinue their drug therapy because they now feel well. If they stop their medication after a few years, they will again lose bone and increase their risk of fracture. The length of treatment is indefinite.

Treatment goals for the prevention of future fractures must be realistic. It has been pointed out that, if medication only prevents further bone loss rather than increasing bone mass dramatically, the risk for fracture is the same as it was before therapy. It is true that the ideal therapy for osteoporosis should reverse the aging process and increase bone mass to a level where the individual is no longer at risk for fracture. This would represent a cure for osteoporosis, but it is not yet available.

However, treatment does reduce the risk for future fracture. A number of studies have shown that there are fewer fractures in patients receiving a variety of antiosteoporotic medications. If you are 65 years old when you have your first osteoporotic fracture and receive no treatment, you may lose as much as an additional 10% of bone in the ensuing decade, greatly increasing your risk for fracture. By preventing this bone loss and avoiding falls and stress to the spine, the likelihood of future fractures may be substantially reduced.

SUMMARY

Treatment of osteoporosis has improved greatly in the last decade. Antiosteoporotic drug treatment reduces the likelihood of future fractures by increasing bone mass or at least by preventing further bone loss. All patients should also be getting an adequate amount of calcium. The FDA has approved both estrogen and calcitonin as effective in treating osteoporosis. Other medications, such as sodium fluoride, are still being investigated. Medical researchers are also administering several medications either in combination or in sequence.

The next chapter makes predictions concerning future research advances.

APPENDIX

Instructions for the Injection of Calcitonin

An Explanation of Calcimar

Calcimar is the brand name for calcitonin, a hormone extracted from salmon. Before you begin to use Calcimar, your doctor will inject a small amount of the drug under the skin of your forearm to determine if you are allergic to it. If you are, the injected area will become red and irritated. The skin test is just a precaution; few people are allergic to Calcimar.

Health care consumers should always ask their physicians about any medication's potential side effects. I am not aware of any serious complications from the use of Calcimar, but minor side effects have been reported. One is a possible increase in the frequency of urination; this should subside after you have taken a few doses of Calcimar. Nausea after a Calcimar injection is another side effect for some people, but it can be practically eliminated by taking the injection at bedtime. Additional side effects reported less frequently are flushes, rashes, vomiting, diarrhea, and cramps.

Preparing for the Injection

The proper dosage of Calcimar is prescribed by your doctor. Insulin syringes are used for the injection, since they are small and very fine. Most people are pleasantly surprised to find that the discomfort of the injection is minimal; the notion of sticking themselves is more difficult, but this usually becomes easier with practice.

Each syringe has lines on it, numbered 1 to 50. If your dose is prescribed as .25 cubic centimeters (cc), then you pull the plunger to the line marked 25 on the syringe. It is important to ignore any reference to the word "units" on the syringe. Calcimar units and insulin units are not the same. Instead, you should be concerned with the number of cc's that correspond to a line on the syringe.

It is comforting to know that there is no danger to you from one dose of too much Calcimar. For example, if one evening you pull the syringe plunger to line 35 instead of line 25, you have taken too much Calcimar. An occasional mistake will not hurt you. However, do take care to learn how to administer the dosage prescribed for you.

Your doctor may prescribe your Calcimar three times a week or once a day. No matter the frequency prescribed, it is useful to devise a system for remembering to take your injections. Some people use a favorite television program as a reminder. Others use a record sheet to keep track of the date of the injection and the site used, which can provide information to your doctor concerning the number of injections you have taken.

Injecting the Calcimar

If you inject Calcimar into a thigh, avoid any area with varicose veins. If you inject the abdomen, place two fingers on either side of the navel and avoid that area.

Use cotton soaked in alcohol or a pre-packaged alcohol swab to cleanse the skin before injecting. Wait a few seconds to let the alcohol dry. If you feel a burning sensation when you inject the Calcimar, you did not let the alcohol dry—the alcohol causes the burning, not the Calcimar. You may leave a spot of blood on your skin after you remove the needle, which is normal.

Injections within the same area should be about 2 inches apart; however, it is better if you rotate injection sites. An example of injection site rotation is Monday, right thigh; Wednesday, left thigh; Friday, right abdomen; Monday, left abdomen; and Wednesday, right thigh.

Steps for Injecting Calcimar

Step 1

Wash your hands. You do not want bacteria or viruses to contaminate your needle, or the injection site.

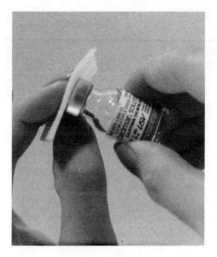

Step 2

Wipe top of bottle with alcohol swab.

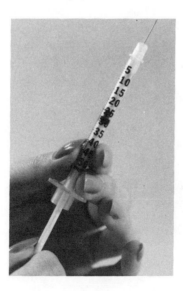

Step 3

Draw air into the syringe by pulling back on the plunger. The amount of air should be equal to the Calcimar dose.

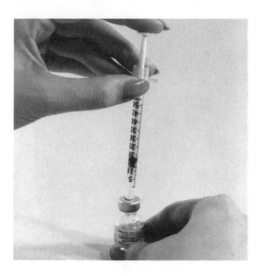

Step 4

With the bottle standing upright, insert the needle into the rubber stopper on the bottle and push the plunger.

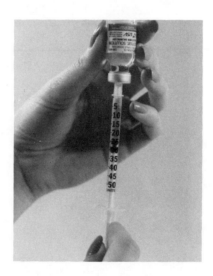

Step 5

Turn the bottle and syringe upside down. Slowly pull the plunger down to the top of the black line that marks your exact dose. Check for air bubbles. The air in the syringe is harmless, however, an air bubble will reduce the amount of Calcimar injected.

Step 6

Remove the needle from the bottle. Cover the needle until you are ready to inject.

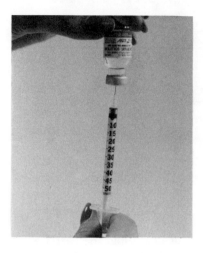

Step 7

When the Calcimar bottle is almost empty, you must reposition the needle; otherwise your syringe will fill with air, not Calcimar. To reposition the needle, you must pull the needle almost out of the vial.

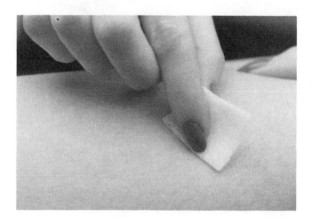

Step 8

Wipe the area where you will inject Calcimar with an alcohol swab. Allow the alcohol to dry.

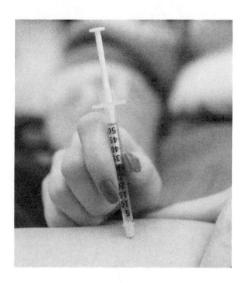

Step 9

Pinch up a large area of skin. Hold the barrel of the syringe like a pencil or dart. Firmly and quickly insert the needle into the muscle to the hub of the needle.

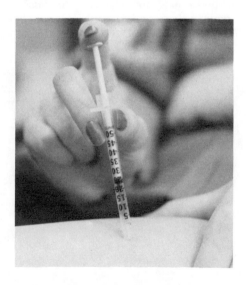

Step 10

Inject the Calcimar by pushing down on the plunger, steadily and gradually.

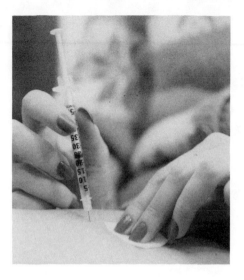

Step 11

Remove the needle quickly and be ready to apply pressure to the area to stop bleeding. Do not rub the area.

Step 12

Using the needle cover, bend the needle back and forth until it breaks.

Additional Tips

Calcimar is a clear liquid packaged in a rubber-stopped vial; each vial will provide four to eight injections, depending on your dose. Always check the expiration date before you make a purchase. Calcimar should be kept refrigerated, but not frozen. If you frequently travel long distances you may want to purchase the Insulin Insulator (about $15.00, available at pharmacies), but a wide-mouth thermos is usually sufficient.

Comparison shopping is probably worthwhile. Calcimar and syringe prices may vary widely. Larger drugstore chains usually have better prices on syringes.

13 CHAPTER

Hope for the Future

The acknowledged father of metabolic disease is Dr. Fuller Albright, who conducted research at Massachusetts General Hospital in Boston in the first half of this century. Dr. Albright studied the balance of calcium and phosphorous in the human body. He carefully controlled his subjects' diets and collected and analyzed their urine and stools for calcium and phosphorus. Although this method seems simple (albeit fastidious) in the space age, much of what we know about osteoporosis today was developed at that time. Dr. Albright defined osteoporosis as a disorder involving too little bone per unit volume. He also recognized the contribution of aging and estrogen deficiency to the development of osteoporosis and was the first to introduce estrogens as treatment.

Many major medical advances have been made since Dr. Albright's time. Calcitonin and calcitriol were unrecognized as viable treatments 50 years ago. Techniques are readily available to measure the minute quantities of hormones in bodily fluids. Researchers have developed quantitative techniques to measure bone mass. However, along with these technological advances has come the high cost of sophisticated research instruments and complex research projects.

Because of its great wealth and commitment, the United States is the world leader in biomedical research. Most of the financial support comes from the budget of the National Institutes of Health (NIH). For specific osteoporosis research, funding has been available from the Institute of Aging and the National Institute of Arthritis, Diabetes, Digestive and Kidney Disease. Unfortunately, the amount of funds available for osteoporosis-related research has not been overwhelming. Moreover, until recently, voluntary groups have made little effort to support osteoporosis research. In general, voluntary groups in the United States have been active in fundraising for research and patient services for a wide variety of chronic illness. The March of Dimes, the Muscular Dystrophy Foundation, the American Cancer Society, the American Heart Association, and the American Diabetes Association are national organizations with local chapters. A foundation even exists for a relatively rare metabolic bone disorder—the Pagets' Disease Foundation. Yet, the National Osteoporosis Foundation has only recently started its work.

I believe that a major reason for the delay in attention to osteoporosis has been the mistaken belief that osteoporosis is an inevitable consequence of aging. Moreover, osteoporosis is not a killer disease like cancer. Finally, the plight of the elderly has not been as appealing a problem for fund-raising as other diseases.

The future of osteoporosis-related research depends to a large extent on the amount of available funding. The annual budget of the NIH for cancer research exceeds $1 billion, whereas funding for osteoporosis is a fraction of this amount. Fortunately, a growing public interest in osteoporosis has led to an increase in funding. In 1987, the NIH provided funds for the establishment of Centers of Excellence in Osteoporosis Research. You can support osteoporosis research by writing to your congressional representative and by donating personal funds to institutes for osteoporosis research. In this way, you can help influence the future.

CURRENT RESEARCH IN OSTEOPOROSIS

The NIH periodically publishes an evaluation of its musculoskeletal disease program that makes specific recommendations for further areas that should receive research support. This section will discuss some of the ongoing research programs and important unanswered questions relating to osteoporosis. I will add those areas that I believe are worthy of further investigation as well as areas that were indicated as important in the April 1984 Consensus Meeting on Osteoporosis and later in the meeting on research held at the NIH in February 1987.

Studies on Risk Assessment and Prevention

The information that has been obtained concerning risk factors for the development of osteoporosis is based on comparison of osteoporotic women with age-matched controls. In the coming years, the relative contributions of each risk factor will be better known.

The bone-mass predictions for who is at risk need to be tested. This will involve long-term studies on large populations of women so that intervention is shown to prevent fractures. From a scientific point of view, although our recommendations for prevention make sense, they must be proven by showing that instituting preventative measures results in a decrease in the incidence of fractures. The NIH is currently supporting a large study that should clarify the role of the various risk factors.

The relative effectiveness of various preventative measures needs to be established. Most important, the value of increasing calcium intake must be more firmly established through clinical trials. Studies on the bioavailability of calcium in supplements, fortified foods, and plant sources must be performed. New methods could be developed to select women who will respond to an increase in calcium intake. In addition, it is unknown whether a program of calcium supplementation and exercise may be as effective as is estrogen replacement in preventing postmenopausal bone loss. The interactions between exercise, estrogen, and nutrition in each phase of the life cycle should be studied. It is not clear how long estrogen replacement must be continued: Are preventative measures such as estrogen and exercise useful after the ages of 60 to 65?

Estrogen-Progestin Therapy

Long-term prospective studies to establish whether estrogen protects against coronary artery disease must be conducted. Transcutaneous systems for the delivery of estrogen should be tested further. The necessity of using progestins is also not fully established. For example, in women who have had a hysterectomy and therefore who are not at risk for endometrial cancer, should progestins still be used? The long-term risks of taking progestins must be established. The safest effective form of hormonal replacement therapy is yet to be developed.

The Effects of Exercise on Bone

The underlying mechanisms at the level of bone cells whereby exercise stimulates bone formation need to be more completely understood. The amount and type of exercise required to prevent bone loss and to attain maximal peak bone mass are yet to be determined. For example, the duration of weight-bearing exercises needs to be determined just as the duration of aerobic exercise for the maintenance of cardiorespiratory fitness is already known. The relative importance of exercise in the different stages of the life cycle must be established.

Clinical Trials for Efficacy of Drug Treatment

The NIH is currently supporting a study to determine the safety and efficacy of fluoride in the treatment of osteoporosis. Efficacy will be established by demonstrating a reduction in the fracture rate. Clinical trials will be performed using the coherence therapy scheme of treatment. New drugs that stimulate bone formation should be developed. Calcitonin will probably become available in a nasal spray so that it does not have to be taken by injection. Chemical modifications in the structure of vitamin D could provide new medications that increase bone mass.

Because osteoporosis is a heterogenous disorder, bone biopsy studies should be performed to determine whether subgroups of patients respond to one form of therapy and not to others. Individualized treatment based on bone biopsy results should be investigated: Should patients with a quiescent biopsy be treated with fluoride to stimulate bone formation, and should patients with high turnover be treated with calcitonin to reduce bone resorption? Noninvasive methods to assess bone turnover (like osteocalcin measurement) will be developed. New methods for treating osteoporosis with medications given in sequence (coherence therapy) will be explored.

Better and Less Expensive Methods for Bone Mass Measurement

The optimal method for screening large populations for low bone mass must be accurate, safe, and inexpensive. New methods for bone-mass measurement should be further refined. The optimal screening procedures with densitometry will be developed in terms of the use of single- or dual-photon absorptiometry and of detecting women with rapid postmenopausal bone loss. New methods that measure bone strength rather than density should be developed.

Understanding Local Control of Bone Cells

Recent studies have shown that bone-cell cultures can be grown and kept alive. As a result it has been possible to examine the effects of hormones and other substances on bone cells. These studies have also identified a number of local factors that control bone remodeling. Much information will be derived from these studies. Most such studies have not been performed on human bone because of technical difficulties, but these difficulties must be overcome so that human rather than rat bone cells can be studied. The study of how new bone is formed may lead to the development of drugs that increase bone mass dramatically.

FUTURE RESEARCH—WHAT DOES THE NEXT DECADE HOLD?

In the next decade, we can expect a number of research accomplishments in the areas of osteoporosis treatment and prevention. Researchers will refine methods for detecting at-risk populations, and more precise recommendations regarding exercise, estrogens, and diet will be forthcoming. We will also see the development of safer forms of hormonal replacement therapy. Physicians will be able to prescribe intranasal calcitonin for women who can't take estrogens. Public intervention on a mass scale will be developed, which should result in a reduction in the incidence of osteoporosis. The next 10 years will establish the efficacy of drug treatment of osteoporosis and will witness the development of new forms of therapy. Undoubtedly, research advances will greatly expand the information we now have, and the future will be much brighter for both the prevention and the treatment of osteoporosis. You can keep abreast of advances by joining the National Osteoporosis Foundation; 1625 Eye Street, N.W.; Suite 1011; Washington, D.C. 20006.

Glossary

Acupuncture: A Chinese medical practice that treats illness by puncturing specified areas of the skin with needles

Aerobic exercise: Exercise in which muscles use oxygen; stimulates the heart and lungs while increasing circulation and improving muscle tone

Alkaline phosphatase: An enzyme that is useful in the recognition of bone activity and diseases of bone

Amenorrhea: The cessation of menstrual periods

Anabolic steroids: Drugs with the same biochemical effect of testosterone but with less of the masculinizing effects

Anaerobic exercise: Different from aerobic exercise in that the muscles do not use oxygen to carry out the exercise (stretching)

Analgesic: An agent that relieves pain

Anorexia nervosa: A condition, usually seen in girls and young women, characterized by severe and prolonged inability or refusal to eat

Antidepressant: Medication that relieves depression

Antihypertensive drugs: Agents that reduce high blood pressure

Anti-inflammatory: Counteracting or suppressing inflammation

Antipsychotic: Medication used in the treatment of psychiatric illness

Arthritis: Inflammation of a joint

Ataxiameter: An apparatus for measuring ataxia (failure of muscular coordination)

Atherosclerosis (hardening of the arteries): A common form of arteriosclerosis in which deposits of yellowish plaques containing cholesterol are formed in the arteries

Atrophy: A wasting away, or a decrease in the size, of a cell, tissue, organ, or other body part

Baroreceptor: A sensory nerve ending that is stimulated by changes in pressure, as those in the walls of blood vessels

Benign: Not malignant, or noncancerous

Bioavailability: Refers to the fact that different forms of the same chemical may produce varied effects, depending on how they are processed

Biofeedback: The process of providing visual or auditory evidence to a person of the status of a body function so that he or she may exert control over the function

Bladder trigone: A smooth triangular portion of the mucous membrane at the base of the bladder

Bone densitometry: Determination of the density of bone by comparison with that of another material

Bursae (singular bursa): Sac or saclike cavities filled with fluid situated in the tissues at which friction (bursitis) would otherwise develop

Calcification: The process of depositing calcium in bone

Calciotropic hormones: Parathyroid hormone, calcitonin, and calcitriol, the hormones that control calcium homeostasis

Calcitonin: A hormone that lowers serum calcium and phosphate levels, inhibits bone resorption, and serves as an antagonist to parathyroid hormone

Calcitriol: The active form of vitamin D that increases calcium absorption

Calisthenic exercise: A system of light gymnastics for promoting strength and flexibility

Cardiac arrhythmia: Any variation from the normal rhythm of the heart

Cardiovascular: Pertaining to the heart and blood vessels

Catecholamines: A group of hormones with different roles in the functioning of the sympathetic and central nervous systems

Cerebrovascular insufficiency: Inadequacy of the blood supply to the brain

Chelated calcium: A form of calcium sold in health-food stores

Climacteric: The decrease of the reproductive period in men and women, culminating in menopause in women

Collagen: A protein that is part of the matrix of bone

Computed Tomography (previously called Computerized Axial Tomography) (CAT): An X ray that, via computer, provides images of the cross section of the body

Conatural supplements: A combination of the synthetic and natural forms of a supplement

Conjugated estrogens: A mixture of several estrogenic compounds

Cortical bone: The dense bone that surrounds the trabecular bone

Cortisol: A hormone produced by the adrenal glands

Crush fracture: A vertebral fracture caused by forces on the spine that compress both the front and the back of a vertebra

Cyclic: Pertaining to or occurring in cycles (not continuously)

Cytologic: Refers to the microscopic structure of cells

D & C (dilatation and curettage): Stretching of the cervix and scraping the wall of the uterus

Diuretics: A drug that increases the volume of urine produced by promoting the excretion of salt and water from the kidneys; commonly known as a "water pill"

Doppler: A test that uses ultrasound to measure blood flow

Double tetracycline labeling: Two types of antibiotics are taken at different times to measure the rate of bone formation on a bone biopsy

Drop attack: An episode in which an individual suddenly falls to the floor

Elemental calcium: The actual amount of calcium in a supplement compound, as opposed to the weight of the entire compound

Endocrine system: Consists of the hypothalamus, pituitary gland, thyroid, pancreas, parathyroid, thymus, adrenal glands, and gonads

Endometrial hyperplasia: The forerunner of cancer of the uterus; characterized by an excess number of cells of the uterine lining

Endometrium: The lining of the uterus

Endorphins: Opiatelike substances released from the brain that reduce pain threshold and produce sedation

Estrogen: The group of steroid hormones (including estriol, estrone, and estradiol) made by the ovaries that control female sexual development and promote the growth and function of the female sex organs and secondary sexual characteristics (such as breast development)

Femur: Thighbone

Fluoridic bone: Bone that contains excess fluoride

Fracture threshold: A theoretical concept that relates bone-mass level to risk for fracture

Gastritis: Stomach irritation

Gluteus maximus: The major buttocks muscles

Gonadal hormones: Estrogen in women and testosterone in men

Gonads: The reproductive glands—ovaries or testes

Herniated disk: A protrusion of a vertebral disk that may impinge on nerve roots

High-density lipoprotein (HDL): Believed to remove cholesterol and to protect against atherosclerosis; commonly known as the "good" cholesterol

Histologic: Refers to the microscopic structure of tissues

Holter monitor: An instrument that records the cardiac rhythm over a 24-hour period

Homeostasis: The physiological process by which the internal systems of the body (e.g., blood pressure, body temperature) are maintained at equilibrium despite variations in external conditions

Humerus: The bone of the upper arm

Hydroxyapatite: The structural part of bone consisting of minerals and water

Hydroxyproline: An amino acid that reflects bone resorption

Hypercalciuria: The presence in the urine of an abnormally high concentration of calcium

Hypercalcemia: High blood calcium level

Hyperparathyroidism: An excess production of parathyroid hormone

Hypertension: High blood pressure

Hyperthyroidism: An excess amount of thyroid hormone

Hypertrophy: An increase in the size of an organ or tissue

Hypogonadism: Abnormally decreased functional activity of the gonads

Hysterectomy: The surgical removal of the uterus

Idiopathic osteoporosis: The description given to the condition in young adults of either sex when the cause is unknown

Imagery: The formation of mental images

Intervertebral disks: The cushionlike material between vertebrae that function like shock absorbers

Involutional melancholia: Severe depression at the time of menopause

Isometric exercise: Exercise in which one muscle or part of the body is pitted against another in forceful but motionless pressing, pushing, pulling, or flexion

Juvenile osteoporosis: Affects prepubescent boys and girls

Kyphosis: Abnormally increased curvature of the thoracic spine (hunchback)

Learned pain syndrome: Refers to patients who have learned to behave in a sick, dependent role and who often are overly dependent on physicians, family, or friends for support

Lipoproteins: A combination of lipid and protein

Low-density lipoprotein (LDL): The protein that carries cholesterol to tissues; also known as the "bad" cholesterol

Lumbar extensor muscles: The muscles located between the thorax and the pelvis

Lumbar lordosis: Abnormally increased curvature of the spine (hollow back, saddle back, swayback)

Lumbar vertebrae: (L1 through L5) The five bones of the spinal column located between the thorax and the sacrum

Lumbosacral: Pertaining to the area of the spine below the thorax

Mammogram: X-ray examination of the breast

Menarche: The age at which the menstrual cycle begins (usually between ages 10 and 14)

Menopause: The natural cessation of menstrual periods that occurs in mid-life, usually between the ages of 45 and 55

Menstruation: Normal uterine bleeding that recurs usually at 4-week intervals

Metabolic bone diseases: Generalized diseases of the bone that affect the entire skeleton (osteoporosis and osteomalacia)

Metacarpals: The bones between the wrist and fingers

Milk-alkali syndrome: Refers to high blood calcium levels, deposits of calcium in tissues outside of bone, and even renal failure caused by consuming large amounts of milk and calcium carbonate (from antacids)

Mineralization: The process of depositing minerals in bone

Modeling: The change in the shape of bones in response to mechanical stress

Multiple myeloma: A malignant neoplasm usually arising in bone marrow

Musculoskeletal: Pertaining to the muscles and bones of the body

Myocardial infarction: Heart attack

Neural arch: The posterior continuation of the vertebral bodies supported by spinal muscles and ligaments

Neutron: Electrically neutral, or uncharged, particle of matter in an atom

Neutron activation analysis: Analysis of the composition of a substance by measuring its interaction with neutrons

Nitroglycerine: A medication that increases the supply of blood to the heart and is used in the treatment of angina pectoris

Nulliparity: Never having given birth to a living child

Oophorectomy: The surgical removal of the ovaries

Orthoses: Orthopedic appliances or apparatus used to support, align, prevent, or correct deformities or to improve the function of movable parts of the body

Osteoarthritis: A disease of the joint cartilage

Osteoblasts: Cells that are responsible for the formation of bone

Osteoclasts: Large cells that break down (dissolve) calcified bone

Osteocytes: Cells (usually within bone rather than on the surface) that may initiate calcification

Osteoid: Unmineralized bone matrix

Osteomalacia: Softening of the bones often caused by a deficiency of vitamin D

Osteosclerosis: Hard or brittle bones

Parathyroid hormone: Controls the movement of calcium and phosphate in the body

Perimenopausal: The period of time around menopause

Periosteal: The outer surface of bone

Phantom: A model of the body

Photon absorptiometry: Measurement of a particle of radiant energy by an instrument after the energy is absorbed by a material such as bone

Physical therapist: A technician trained in the treatment and prevention of disease with the aid of physical agents such as light, heat, cold, water, and electricity or of mechanical apparatus

Placebo: A pill that has no active ingredients

Postmenopausal osteoporosis: Occurs in women within 15 to 20 years after menopause

Postural hypotension: A drop in blood pressure caused by a change in position

Primary osteoporosis: Diagnosed when it has been determined that the osteoporosis is not linked to another illness

Progesterone: A hormone produced by the ovaries following ovulation

Progestins: Natural or synthetic compounds having similar effects to progesterone

Proprioceptive signals: Sensory nerve signals that give information concerning movements and position of the body

Protein electrophoresis: A test that separates the variety of proteins in the blood or urine; used to detect multiple myeloma

Proteinuria: Presence of excess protein in the urine

Psychotropic drugs: Medication that affects the mental state

Pulmonary: Pertaining to the lungs

Pulmonary embolism: The sudden blocking of an artery by a clot that has been carried by the blood to the lungs

Quantitative: Exact

Quantitative digital radiography: An improved form of densitometry

RDA: Recommended dietary allowance

Radiographic morphometry: Measurement of bone thickness using X rays

Radiologist: A physician specializing in the use of radioactive substances and X ray in the diagnosis and treatment of disease

Radiolucency: The degree of lightness on an X ray

Radius: The bone of the outer, or thumb side, of the forearm

Remodeling: The dissolution and formation of bone

Resorption: The dissolution of bone

Scoliosis: Curvature of the spine

Screening: Testing a large number of people for a disease

Secondary osteoporosis: Diagnosed when the osteoporosis is linked to another illness

Sedentary: Inactive

Senile or involutional osteoporosis: Used primarily to describe steoporosis in the elderly

Sleep deprivation syndrome: Symptoms that result from a lack of sleep such as fatigue, irritability, and difficulty concentrating

Spinal flexion: Bending forward at the waist

Syncope: A temporary loss of consciousness

TENS: Transcutaneous electrical nerve stimulation to relieve pain

Testosterone: The principal male sex hormone; made by the testes

Thiazide: Diuretics that inhibit the reabsorption of sodium by the kidney and also decrease the urinary excretion of calcium

Thoracic vertebrae: (D1 through D12) The 12 bones of the spinal column to which the ribs attach

Thoracolumbar junction: The junction of the thoracic and the lumbar spine

Trabeculae: Struts of trabecular bone on the vertebrae that are organized to withstand stress on the spine

Trabecular bone: The part of the bone that is in contact with bone marrow

Transdermal: Through the skin

Transport: The movement of a substance into or out of cells either actively or passively

Type I osteoporosis: Results from postmenopausal bone loss

Type II osteoporosis: Occurs in older individuals

Ulna: The inner, larger bone of the forearm opposite the radius

Urethra: The canal that conveys urine from the bladder to outside the body

Urogenital: Pertaining to the urinary and genital apparatus

Vagina: The canal in the female, extending from the vulva to the cervis uteri, that receives the penis during sexual intercourse

Vasomotor flushes: Affecting the diameter of a blood vessel to cause transient redness of the face and neck

Vertebrae: Any of the 33 bones of the spinal column

Vertigo: A disabling sensation in which the affected individual feels that he or she or the surroundings are spinning

Vulva: The region of the external genital organs of the female

Wedge fracture: A vertebral fracture caused by forces on the spine that compress the front of a vertebra more than the back

References

Albright, F. (1947). The effect of hormones on osteogenesis in man. *Recent Progress in Hormone Research, 1*, 293-353.

Aloia, J.F. (1981). Exercise and skeletal health. *Journal of the American Geriatric Society, 29*(3), 104-107.

Aloia, J.F., Cohn, S.H., Babu, T., Abesamis, C., Kalici, N., & Ellis, K. (1978). Skeletal mass and body composition in marathon runners. *Metabolism: Clinical and Experimental, 27*, 1793-1796.

Aloia, J.F., Cohn, S.H., Ostuni, J.A., Cane, R., & Ellis, K. (1978). Prevention of involutional bone loss by exercise. *Annals of Internal Medicine, 89*, 356-358.

Aloia, J.F., Cohn, S.H., Vaswani, A., Yeh, J.K., Yuen, K., & Ellis, K. (1985). Risk factors for postmenopausal osteoporosis. *American Journal of Medicine, 78*, 95-100.

Aloia, J.F., Kapoor, A., Vaswani, A., & Cohn, S.H. (1981). Changes in body composition following therapy of osteoporosis with methandrostenolone. *Metabolism: Clinical and Experimental, 30*, 1076-1079.

Aloia, J.F., Vaswani, A., Kapoor, A., Yeh, J.K., & Cohn, S.H. (1985). Treatment of osteoporosis with calcitonin, with and without growth hormone. *Metabolism: Clinical and Experimental, 34*, 124-129.

Aloia, J.F., Vaswani, A., Yeh, J.K., & Cohn, S.H. (1988). Premenopausal bone mass is related to physical activity. *Archives of Internal Medicine, 148*, 121-123.

Aloia, J.F., Vaswani, A.N., Yeh, J.K., Yasumura, S., & Cohn, S.H. (1988). Calcitriol in the treatment of postmenopausal osteoporosis. *American Journal of Medicine, 84*, 401-408.

Aloia, J.F., Zanzi, I., Ellis, K., Jowsey, J., Roginsky, M.S., Wallach, S., & Cohn, S.H. (1976). Effects of growth hormone in osteoporosis. *Journal of Clinical Endocrinology & Metabolism, 54*, 992-999.

Aloia, J.F., Zanzi, I., Vaswani, A., Ellis, K. & Cohn, S.H. (1982). Combination therapy for osteoporosis with estrogen, fluoride and calcium. *Journal of the American Geriatric Society*, **30**(1), 13-17.

Bain, C., Willett, W., Hennekens, C., Rosner, B., Bilanger, C., & Speizer, S.E. (1981). Use of postmenopausal hormones and risk of myocardial infarction. *Circulation*, **64**(1), 42-46.

Bell, N.H., Greene, A., Epstein, S., Oxemann, M.J., Shaw, S., & Shary, I. (1976). Evidence for alteration of the vitamin D-endocrine system in blacks. *Journal of Clinical Investigation*, **76**(2), 470-473.

Black-Sandler, R., LaPorte, R.E., Sashin, D., Kuller, L.H., Sternglass, E., Cauley, J.A., & Link, M.M. (1982). Determinants of bone mass in menopause. *Preventive Medicine*, **11**, 269-280.

Brocklehurst, J.C., Exton-Smith, A.N., Lempert-Barber, S.M., Hunt, L.P., & Palmer, M.K. (1978). Fracture of the femur in old age: A two-centre study of associated clinical factors and the cause of the fall. *Age and Aging*, **7**, 7-15.

Campbell, A.J., Reinken, J., Allan, B.C., & Martinez, G.S. (1981). Falls in old age: A study of frequency and related clinical factors. *Age and Aging*, **10**, 264-270.

Chesnut, C.H., Nelp, W.B., & Baylink, D.J. (1977). Effects of methandrostenolone on postmenopausal bone wasting as assessed by changes in total bone mineral mass. *Metabolism: Clinical and Experimental*, **26**(3), 267-277.

Council on Scientific Affairs. (1983). Estrogen replacement in the menopause. *Journal of the American Medical Association*, **249**, 359-361.

Ettinger, B., Genant, H., & Cann, C. (1987). Postmenopausal bone loss is prevented by treatment with low-dosage estrogen with calcium. *Annals of Internal Medicine*, **106**, 40-45.

Frost, H.M. (1979). Treatment of osteoporosis by manipulation of coherent bone cell populations. *Clinical Orthopaedics and Related Research*, **143**, 227-244.

Gryfe, C.I., Amies, A., & Ashley, M.J. (1977). A longitudinal study of falls in an elderly population: I. Incidence and morbidity. *Age and Aging*, **6**, 201-210.

Heaney, R.P., & Recker, R.R. (1986). Distribution of calcium absorption in middle-age women. *American Journal of Clinical Nutrition*, **43**, 299-305.

Heaney, R.P., Recker, R.R., & Saville, P.D. (1977). Calcium balance and calcium requirements in middle-age women. *American Journal of Clinical Nutrition*, **30**, 1603-1611.

Hillner, B.E., Hollenberg, J.P., & Pauker, S.G. (1986). Postmenopausal estrogens in prevention of osteoporosis: Benefit virtually without risk if cardiovascular effects are considered. *American Journal of Medicine*, **80**, 1115-1127.

Horsman, A., Gallagher, J.C., Simpson, M., & Nordin, B.E.C. (1977). Prospective trial of estrogen and calcium in postmenopausal women. *British Medical Journal*, **2**, 789-792.

Jensen, J., Christiansen, C., & Rodbro, P. (1985). Cigarette smoking, serum estrogens, and bone loss during hormone-replacement therapy early after menopause. *New England Journal of Medicine*, **313**(16), 973-975.

Jick, H., Dinian, B., & Rothman, K.J. (1978). Noncontraceptive estrogens and nonfatal myocardial infarction. *Journal of the American Medical Association*, **239**, 1407-1408.

MacDonald, P.C. (1981). Editorial: Estrogen plus progestin in postmenopausal women. *New England Journal of Medicine*, **305**, 1644-1645.

Matkovic, V., Kastial, K., Simonovic, I., Buzina, R., Bordarec, A., & Nordin, B.E.C. (1979). Bone status and fracture rates in two regions in Yugoslavia. *American Journal of Clinical Nutrition*, **32**, 540-549.

Mazzuoli, G.F., Passeri, M., Gennari, C., Minisola, S., Antonelli, R., Vallarta, C., Palummeri, E., Corvellin, G.F., Gonnelli, S., & Francini, G. (1986). Effects of salmon calcitonin in postmenopausal osteoporosis: A controlled double-blind clinical study. *Calcified Tissue International*, **38**, 3-8.

Melton, L.J. III, & Riggs, B.L. (1983). Epidemiology of age-related fractures. In A.V. Avioli (Ed.), *The Osteoporotic syndrome: Detection, prevention and treatment* (pp. 45-72). New York: Grune & Stratton.

Nilas, L., Christiansen, C., & Rodbro, P. (1984). Calcium supplementation and postmenopausal bone loss. *British Medical Journal*, **289**(6452), 1103-1106.

Nilsson, B.E., & Westlin, N.E. (1971). Bone density in athletes. *Clinical Orthopaedics and Related Research*, **77**, 179-182.

Overstall, P.W. (1980). Prevention of falls in the elderly. *Journal of the American Geriatric Society*, **28**, 481-484.

Overstall, P.W., Exton-Smith, A.N., Imms, F.J., & Johnson, A.L. (1977). Falls in the elderly related to postural imbalance. *British Medical Journal*, **1**(6056), 261-264.

Padwick, M.L., Pryse-Davies, J., & Whitehead, M.I. (1986). A simple method for determining the optimal dosage of progestin in postmenopausal women receiving estrogens. *New England Journal of Medicine*, **315**, 930-934.

Recker, R.R., Saville, P.D., & Heaney, R.P. (1977). The effect of estrogens and calcium carbonate on bone loss in post-menopausal women. *Annals of Internal Medicine,* **87**, 649-655.

Reeve, J., Meunier, P.J., Parsons, J.A., Bernat, M., Bijvoet, O.L.M., Courpron, P., Edouard, C., Klenerman, L., Neer, R.M., Renier, J.C., Slovik, D., Vismans, F.J.F.E., & Potts, J. (1980). Anabolic effect of human parathyroid hormone fragment on trabecular bone in involutional osteoporosis. *British Medical Journal,* **280**, 1340-1344.

Riggs, B.L., Seeman, E., Hodgson, S.F., Taves, D.R., & O'Fallon, W.M. (1982). Effect of the fluoride/calcium regimen on vertebral fracture occurrence in postmenopausal osteoporosis: Comparison with conventional therapy. *New England Journal of Medicine,* **306**, 446.

Riggs, B.L., Wahner, H.W., Seeman, E., Offord, K.P., Dunn, W.L., Mazess, R.B., Johnson, K.A., & Melton, L.J. III (1982). Changes in bone mineral density of the proximal spine and femur with aging. Differences between the postmenopausal and senile osteoporosis syndromes. *Journal of Clinical Investigation,* **70**, 716-732.

Riis, B., Thomsen, K., & Christiansen, C. (1987). Does calcium supplementation prevent postmenopausal bone loss?: A double-blind, controlled clinical study. *New England Journal of Medicine,* **316**(4), 173-177.

Ross, R., Paganini-Hill, A., & Mack, T. (1981). Menopausal estrogen therapy and protection from death from ischemic heart disease. *Lancet,* **1**, 858-860.

Sharkey, B.J. (1984). *Physiology of fitness.* Champaign, IL: Human Kinetics.

Sinaki, M., & Mikkelsen, B.A. (1984). Postmenopausal spinal osteoporosis: Flexion versus extension exercises. *Archives of Physical Medicine and Rehabilitation,* **65**, 593-596.

Smith, E.L., Reddan, W., & Smith, P.E. (1981). Physical activity and calcium modalities for bone mineral increase in aged women. *Medical Science in Sports and Exercise,* **13**, 60-64.

Tobias, J.S., Nayak, L., & Hoehler, F. (1981). Visual perception of verticality and horizontality among elderly fallers. *Archives of Physical Medicine and Rehabilitation,* **62**(12), 619-622.

Warren, M.P., Brooks-Gunn, J., Hamilton, L.H., Warren, L.F., & Hamilton, W.G. (1986). Scoliosis and fractures in young ballet dancers: Relationship to delayed menarche and secondary amenorrhea. *New England Journal of Medicine,* **314**(21), 1348-1353.

Wilmoth, S.K. (1988). *Y's Way to Better Aerobics.* Champaign, IL: Human Kinetics.

Index

Numbers in italics refer to figure numbers.

A

Absorptiometry. *See* Diagnostic testing, Testing
Accidents (tripping), 44
Aerobic exercise, 28, 30, 132, 133
Alcohol, 80, 105
Amenorrhea, 6, 33
Androgens, 197
Antacids, 35
Anticonvulsants, 35
Arthritis, 160, 185
  osteo, 15
  rheumatoid, 27
Ataxiameter, 45
Atherosclerosis, 27, 117

B

Balance, loss of, 4
Baroreceptors (pressure detectors), 45
Bending techniques, 42
Biopsy
  bone, 171
  endometrium, 116, 173
Black race, 25, 29
Body image, 182-183
Bone
  calcification of, 11
  cortical, 10
  density, *2.10*
  fluoridic, 37
  formation, 3-4
  gain, 19-20
  loss, 19-20, 22
  mass, *2.8, 3.1*
  measurement of, 214
  mineralization (calcification), 11
  modeling, 9, 14
  as organs, 14-16
  radius, 17
  remodeling, 3, 38
  resorption, 4
  strength, 37-38
  trabecular, 10
Bone cells
  control of, 214
  osteoblasts, 12
  osteoclasts, 12
  osteocytes, 12
Bone mass, *2.8, 2.9*
  activity, 29-30
  drugs' effects on, 34
  estrogen, 31-33
  heredity, 28
  hormones, 33
  hypertrophy, 29
  illness effects on, 34
  inactivity effects on, 29-30
Braces, 178-180

C

Caffeine, 28, 30, 104
Calcitonin, 4-5, 33, 198
  injections, 203-209
  nasal spray, 214
Calcitriol, 4-5, 31, 33, 196, 201
Calcium
  absorption, 3
  balance, 7

Calcium (continued)
  "craze," 53-69
  intake, 55, 86, 97-98
  Recommended Dietary Allow-
    ance (RDA) of, 53, 54, 95-97
Calcium homeostasis, 2-7
  endocrine system, 4-7
  gastrointestinal system, 3
  skeletal system, 3
  urinary system, 3
Calcium supplements, 57-64, 98
  bioavailability of, 65-66
  elemental, 64
  harmful, 67
  mineral and vitamins, 66-67
  progestins with, 126
  when to take, 67
Calcium transport, 3
Cancer, 116, 213
  breast, 120, 124, 128, 129
  endometrial (uterine), 118-120,
    123-125
Cane, 48
Cerebrovascular insufficiency, 45
Cholesterol, 73
Cigarette smoking, 28, 34, 118
Collagen, 10
Contraceptives, oral, 19

D

Dairy products
  calcium content of, 81-92
  caloric content of, 93-94
  fat content of, 93-94
Dependency, 182
Diagnostic testing, 157-174
  bone mass measurement,
    157-158
  computed tomography (CAT),
    162
  dual-photon absorptiometry,
    159
  radiographic morphometry, 158
  single-photon absorptiometry,
    159
  total-body neutron activation
    analysis and whole-body
    counting, 158-159

Diet
  and alcohol, 80, 105
  and calcium, 90-92
  eating guide for, 74-78
  and fat, 73
  and fiber, 79
  and sodium, 79
  and starch, 79
  and sugar, 79
  and vitamin A, 105
  and vitamin C, 105
  and vitamin D, 31, 100-102
Dietary goals, 71-72
Dietary guidelines, 72-73
Diets
  for adolescents, 31
  for elderly, 31
  low-calorie, 31
  high-calcium, low-calorie,
    109-114
  saturated fat in, 73
  vegetarian, 105-106
  weight loss, 105-106
Diuretics, 4, 34, 35, 66
Drop attack, 41, 44-45
Drugs, 187-191
  activators, 195
  analgesics, 180, 188, 190
  androgen, 197
  antacids, 55, 58, 65, 67
  anticonvulsants, 35
  antihypertensive, 45
  calcitonin, 203-209
  calcium absorption, 196, 201
  diuretics, 4, 34, 35, 66
  estrogen, 197
  fluoride, 199
  gonadal steroids, 197
  to increase bone formation, 199
  inhibitors, 195
  narcotics, 187
  new, 195
  progestins, 7, 123-126, 213
  steroids, 197
  thyroid hormone, 34, 35
Drug therapy, 192-209, 214
  classification, 195-196

combination therapy, 196, 200
sequential therapy, 196

E

Estrogen, 4, 31-33, 55, 197
American Medical Association
Council recommendations, 120-
121
benefits of, 116
and cancer, 118-120, 123-125.
See also Cancer
controversy, 115-130
and heart attack, 117-118
indications for, 128-129
and menopausal problems, 116
progestin therapy with, 213
replacement therapy, 121-123
risks of, 118-120
transdermal, 123-127
Exercise
effects of, 29, 213-214
goals of, 135
precautions for, 136
preventive program of, 137-146
Exercise, types of
abdominal strengthening, 153
aerobic, 132-133
anaerobic, 133
back extensions, 140, 152
calisthenic, 133
front leg stretch, 143
gentle prone lift, 154
gluteus, 155
head up, 153
heel raisers, 142
isometric, 133
jumping jack, 139
knee bends, 139, 141
leg raise, 154
lower back stretch, 141
pectoral stretching, 152
position control, 144-145, 151
recommendations, 135-138
shoulder-chest stretch, 143
side stretch, 144
situps, 140
skeletal health, 131-156
stand tall, 138, 149, 155

stationary bicycle, 152
strengthening, 132-133
wall arch, 150
Exercise program, 134-136
for elderly, 146-147
for osteoporotic women, 147-
156

F

Falls
causes of, 44
drop attacks, 41, 44-45
preventing, 42, 46
risk of, 43
syncope, 41
Fashion suggestions, 183
Fear of dependency, 182
Femur, 18-19
bone loss in, 22
periosteal diameter of, 38
Fiber, 104
Fluoride, 199
Foods
calcium content of, 81-85, 99
checklist of, for calcium content, 87-92
calcium enriched, 94-95
calcium intake through, 80
cholesterol content of, 81-85
Fracture threshold, 20
Fractures, 1-2
avoiding, 180
Colles', 1, 18, 41
compression, 177
fear of future, 181
grieving process, 180-181
of hip (intertrochanteric), 18, 41
and posture, 178
prevention of, 52
psychological adjustment to,
180-183
of radius, 17-18
rehabilitation of, 175-184
repair of, 37-38
sexual adjustment to, 181
of spine, 41
stress, 41
wedge, 17

G
Gallbladder disease, 27, 120, 129
Glucocorticoids, 35
Gonadal hormones, 5, 7, 20

H
Heredity, 28
High-density lipoproteins (HDL), 73, 117
Hope for the future, 211-215
Hormones
  calciotropic, 4
  Calcitonin, 4-5, 33, 198, 203-209, 214
  calcitriol, 4-5
  catecholamines, 45
  cortisol, 33
  estrogen, 31-33, 55, 197
  gonadal, 5-7, 19
  gonadotropin, 35
  growth hormone, 4, 33
  parathyroid hormone, 4-5, 25
  progestins, 7, 123-126, 213
  testosterone, 6, 125
  thyroid, 34, 35
Holter monitor, 45
Hot flashes, 117
Hunchback. *See* Kyphosis
Hypercalcemia, 5
Hyperparathyroidism, 27
Hyperthyroidism, 34
Hypogonadism, 125
Hysterectomy, 32

I
Immobilization, 27, 29
Insomnia, 117
Isoniazide, 35

K
Kyphosis (hunchback), 177

L
Lactose, 102
  intolerance to, 94
Lifting techniques, 42, 49
Liver disease, 27, 129

M
Mammogram, 126
Menarche, 6

Menopause, 6
  early, 28
  management of, 125-127
  perimenopause, 6
  postmenopause, 6
Menstruation, 7
Metabolic bone disease, 12
Minerals, 102

N
National Institutes of Health, 54, 56, 212
National Osteoporosis Foundation, 212, 215
Nutrition, 30-31, 71-114
  labeling, 95-97
Nutritional myths, 106

O
Obesity, 119
Oophorectomy, 32
Osteoarthritis, 15
Osteomalacia, 9, 12, 37
Osteoporosis
  classification of, 23
  definition of, 1
  genetic influence on, 29
  idiopathic, 23
  involutional, 24
  juvenile, 23
  postmenopausal, 24
  prevention and risk assessment of, 212
  primary, 23
  routes to, 20-22
  secondary, 23
  Type I, 24-25
  Type II, 24-25
Osteosclerosis, 9
Oxalates, 104

P
Pain, 176-177
  chronic, causes of, 185
  clinic, 190-191
  from muscle-spasm, 190
Pain, treatment methods for, 185-191
  acupuncture, 189
  biofeedback, 189

drugs, 187-191
  narcotics, 187
  non-narcotic drugs, 188
  psychoactive drugs, 188
  TENS (transcutaneous electrical
    neuro stimulation), 189
Parathyroid hormone, 4-5
Positional sway, 45
Postural hypotension, 44
Posture, 42, 48, 49, 178
Progestins, 7, 123-126, 213
Proprioceptive signals, 45
Protein, 28

Q
Quackery, 106

R
Radius, 17, 67
  and bone loss, 22
Recommended Dietary Allowance
    (RDA) labeling, 53, 54, 95-97
Research, 212
Risk factors, 27-29
  modifiable, 27-28
  nonmodifiable, 28-29

S
Safety tips, household, 47
Scoliosis, 27, 33
Skeleton
  healthy and osteoporotic, 9-26
  tissue, 10-12
Spinal injury
  avoidance of, 48-50
  devoid of, 50
Spine, 15-17
  bone loss from, 22
  crush fracture of, 16-17
  intervertebral disks, 16
  lumbar, 15
  neural arch, 16
  thoracic vertebrae, 15, 16
  trabeculae, 16
  wedge fracture, 17
Surgical menopause. See Oopho-
    rectomy
Syncope, 41

T
Testes
  hypogonadism, 125
  testosterone, 6, 125
Testing
  blood tests, 169-170
  bone biopsy, 171
  bone densitometry, 167
  bone mass measurement, 157-
    158
  bone scan, 170
  chem-screen, 169
  complete blood count (CBC),
    169
  computed tomography (CAT),
    162
  densitometry, 162
  dual-photon absorptiometry,
    159
  endometrial biopsy, 116, 173
  expense, 165-166
  measuring, 163
  neutron activation analysis, 158
  preferable techniques, 164
  radiation exposure, 164
  radiographic morphometry, 158
  screening, 167-168
  single-photon absorptiometry,
    159
  total body neutron activation,
    158
  urine, 170
  X-ray, 171
Tetracycline, 35
Thyroid Stimulating Hormone
    (TSH), 34
Thyrotoxicosis, 27
Treatment, drugs, 214
Tripping or slipping, 41, 43
Tums, 55, 58, 65, 67

U
United States Recommended
    Dietary Allowance, 95-97

V
Vitamin A, 105
Vitamin C, 105
Vitamin D, 31, 100-102, 109, 201

About the Author

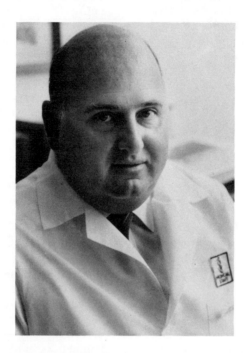

Dr. John Aloia received his doctor of medicine degree from Creighton Medical School in Omaha, Nebraska. He is chairman of the Department of Medicine and director of the Division of Endocrinology and Metabolism at Winthrop-University Hospital in Mineola, New York. Dr. Aloia also serves as associate dean and professor of medicine at the State University of New York at Stony Brook. In addition to his hospital and university responsibilities, Dr. Aloia is very active in many medical organizations and associations, including the American Society for Bone and Mineral Research.

Dr. Aloia has spent many years researching osteoporosis and its effects on women. His research covers such areas as the treatment of osteoporosis with sodium fluoride, estrogen, and calcium; skeletal mass in postmenopausal women; and prevention of bone loss by physical exercise. In addition to *Osteoporosis: A Guide to Prevention and Treatment,* he has published extensively on the subjects of osteoporosis and the loss of bone mass.

Dr. Aloia and his wife Elvira have four children, Maria, John, Mark, and Linda. In his leisure hours, he enjoys spending time with his family and listening to classical music and opera.